overcoming
functional neurological symptoms

a five areas approach

overcoming
functional neurological symptoms
a five areas approach

Professor Chris Williams Professor of Psychosocial Psychiatry and Honorary Consultant Psychiatrist, Academic Unit of Mental Health and Wellbeing, Institute of Health and Wellbeing, University of Glasgow, Glasgow, UK

Catriona Kent
Nurse Consultant, NHS Greater Glasgow and Clyde, UK

Dr Sharon Smith
Royal Edinburgh Hospital, Edinburgh, UK

Dr Alan Carson
Consultant Neuropsychiatrist, Department of Rehabilitation Medicine, Astley Ainslie Hospital, and Department of Clinical Neurosciences, Western General Hospital, Edinburgh. Senior Lecturer, University of Edinburgh, Edinburgh, UK

Professor Michael Sharpe
Psychological Medicine Research, University of Edinburgh, Royal Edinburgh Hospital, Edinburgh, UK

Dr Jonathan Cavanagh
Academic Unit of Mental Health and Wellbeing, Institute of Health and Wellbeing, University of Glasgow, Glasgow UK

Helping you to help yourself

www.livinglifetothefull.com
www.fiveareas.com
www.fiveareasonline.com

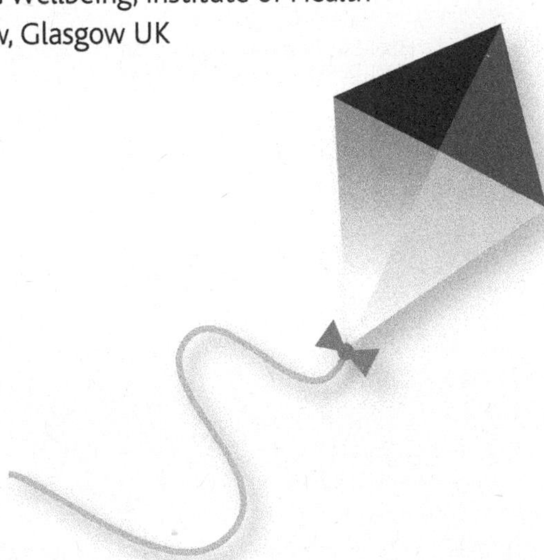

Routledge
Taylor & Francis Group
LONDON AND NEW YORK

First published 2011 by Hodder Arnold

Published 2017 by Routledge
2 Park Square, Milton Park, Abingdon, Oxon OX14 4RN
52 Vanderbilt Avenue, New York, NY 10017

Routledge is an imprint of the Taylor & Francis Group, an informa business

ISBN-13: 978-1-4441-3834-4 (pbk)
ISBN-13: 978-1-138-44543-7 (hbk)

Clinical/teaching licence

Contents

Introduction

Welcome to *Overcoming Unexplained Neurological Symptoms: A Five Areas Approach*. Facing the challenge of how to cope with chronic illness can be difficult, confusing and distressing. Symptoms themselves may interfere and prevent people living life as they wish to. These may include symptoms such as paralysis or weakness, seizures, numbness, slurred speech or altered vision, hearing or speech. There may be symptoms such as pain, tiredness, anxiety or low mood. Sometimes there is a clear cause for symptoms, however sometimes the cause may be unexplained – and so the symptoms are described as *functional* in nature.

A diagnosis of functional neurological symptoms is much more common than you might think. Research in four major neurological centres suggests that about one in three people attending neurology outpatient clinics have this diagnosis. The diagnosis of functional neurological symptoms can be made as accurately as any other diagnosis. The diagnosis usually means that further tests are not required.

Functional symptoms significantly affect how the sufferer lives their life. We now know a lot more than before about the causes of such symptoms, and how to help tackle them. The treatment package described in these workbooks, and the accompanying toolbox, is designed to help you overcome your symptoms. A research study funded by the Medical Research Council has found that the content of this course can be an effective treatment for people with functional neurological symptoms.

This book is designed to actively help you to:

- Learn important information about how functional neurological symptoms can affect your life.
- Work out why you are feeling as you do.
- Learn and practise some practical skills to help change how you feel.

By following the clearly described tools in these workbooks, and the accompanying toolbox, you can make helpful changes to your life.

Who are the workbooks and toolbox for?

You may be using the workbooks for yourself, or perhaps you are a close friend or family member wanting to know more about functional neurological symptoms and how to help. Many healthcare practitioners also use the workbooks in this series to support those they work with.

Self-help approaches can be used by people with problems ranging from mild distress through to more severe symptoms. The key thing is that you feel *able* to use the materials and *want* to use this approach.

Using the workbooks and toolbox

The course involves *reading* the course workbooks and also *working* on problems by putting into practice the things you are learning. Picking the right time to do the course is important. For example, if your concentration, energy or motivation levels are far lower than usual, you may find it very hard to keep your mind on things or to make changes. Other approaches may be more appropriate first – allowing you to come back to use the workbooks and toolbox at a time when you are able to get the most from them. If you find that you are struggling to use the workbooks, or you feel worse as you work through them, please discuss this with your doctor or other healthcare practitioner. The course is not meant to replace getting the right level of support for more severe health problems.

Which workbook should you use first?

There is no right or wrong way to use the workbooks. Many people find it helpful to first read the workbooks in Part 1 (Workbook 1: Introduction. Understanding how people respond to symptoms and Workbook 2: Your brain and body, and how these link to symptoms).

These workbooks will give you a good overview of the approach and will also help you to then move onto the 'Making changes' workbooks in Part 2 of the book. You can use as many or as few workbooks in the course as you wish. You will feel most motivated to try to make changes if you use the workbooks that tackle problems you have noticed in your life and that you want to change.

The third part of the book is the Toolbox, which will help you put all that you have learned in the previous workbooks into practice.

KEY POINT

The key to creating change in your life is *using* the workbooks and *putting what you learn into practice*.

Getting help from others

It can be hard making changes when you feel ground down or stressed. Many people start off trying to improve things with lots of motivation. But feeling ill can sometimes make us quickly give up on change. That's entirely normal and is very human (think how hard people find it keeping New Year resolutions even when they aren't feeling worried about things).

Time and time again, people using resources like this have found the benefits of working with someone else to support and encourage them when things feel hard. We therefore suggest that you partner with someone to help you as you use the course. For example, a health or social services worker, your doctor, a voluntary sector worker or a trusted family member or friend.

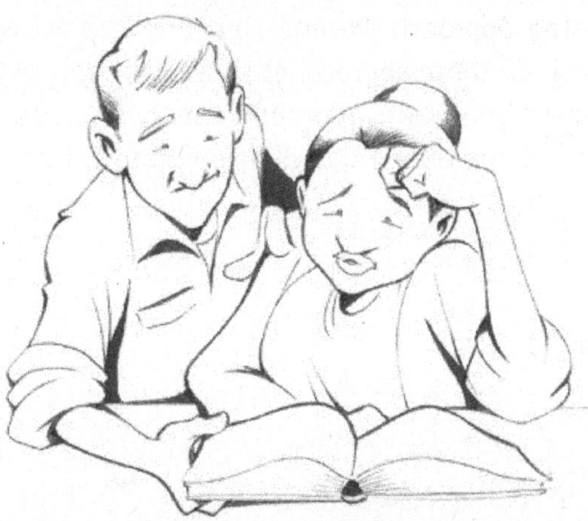

The important thing is to have someone else there, helping you, discussing problems that seem hard – and to say well done when things move forwards.

A word of encouragement

The content of these workbooks and toolbox is based on the cognitive behavioural therapy (CBT; a kind of talking treatment) approach. The developers of CBT have found many effective ways of tackling the common symptoms and problems people face when feeling low.

This course is written in a way that clearly explains what to do, so that you can test the effect of these different suggestions in your own life. The workbooks aim to help you to **regain a sense of control** over how you feel.

The self-help approach can really work

Research has been done on people who use books like this one based on CBT. A research study on this book has shown that when offered with support it can help people experiencing functional neurological symptoms. The course can make a big difference if you can commit to using it.

Making a commitment

Sometimes making changes is easier said (or written) than done. All of us feel discouraged and overwhelmed from time to time. This is even more likely when you feel distressed, anxious, tense or low.

Therefore, **try to make a commitment to use this course** and to keep at it even if you feel discouraged or stuck for some time. To do this you will need to **pace yourself** by using a step-by-step approach. Having someone else to encourage you is also important. The research on these approaches shows just how helpful this can be. Also, be realistic. Bear in mind your motivation and energy levels so that you don't try to do more than you can at one time. This will help you to get as much from the course as you can.

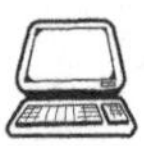

New online resources

An online resource is available to support users of the course: **www.livinglifetothefull.com**. This free website contains short talks that help you to build upon the course workbooks. There is also a moderated chat room where people can swap ideas, hints and tips, as well as offering and receiving mutual support. If you don't have a computer, try to use one in an internet café, or in a public library. Sign up for the free reminder letters there to help you keep on track. You can also freely access TV-based versions of the course from the website. Some people like to see and hear how other people have applied what they have learned. Again, using the site with support and encouragement from someone can be a big help to getting the most out of the approach.

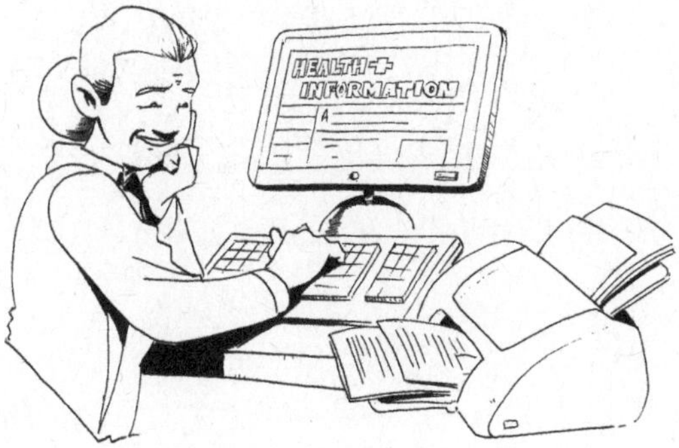

A note about copyright

Acknowledgements

The illustrations in the workbooks have been produced by Keith Chan, kchan75@ hotmail.com. Copies are available as a separate download for clinical use at www. fiveareas.com.

Chris Williams, Catriona Kent, Sharon Smith, Alan Carson, Michael Sharpe and Jonathan Cavanagh

July 2011

Part 1
Understanding how people respond to symptoms

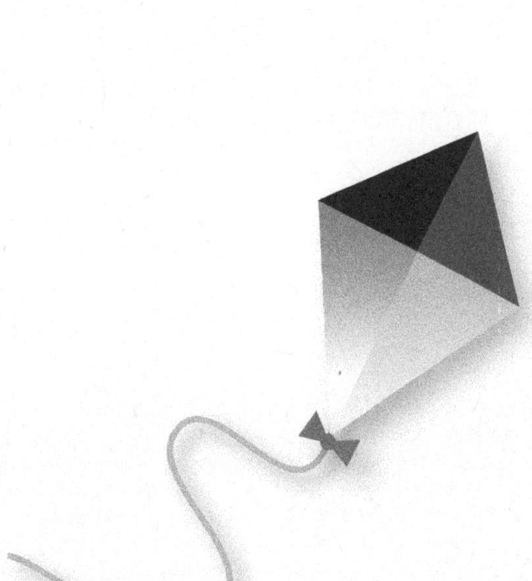

Workbook 1: Introduction

Understanding how people respond to symptoms

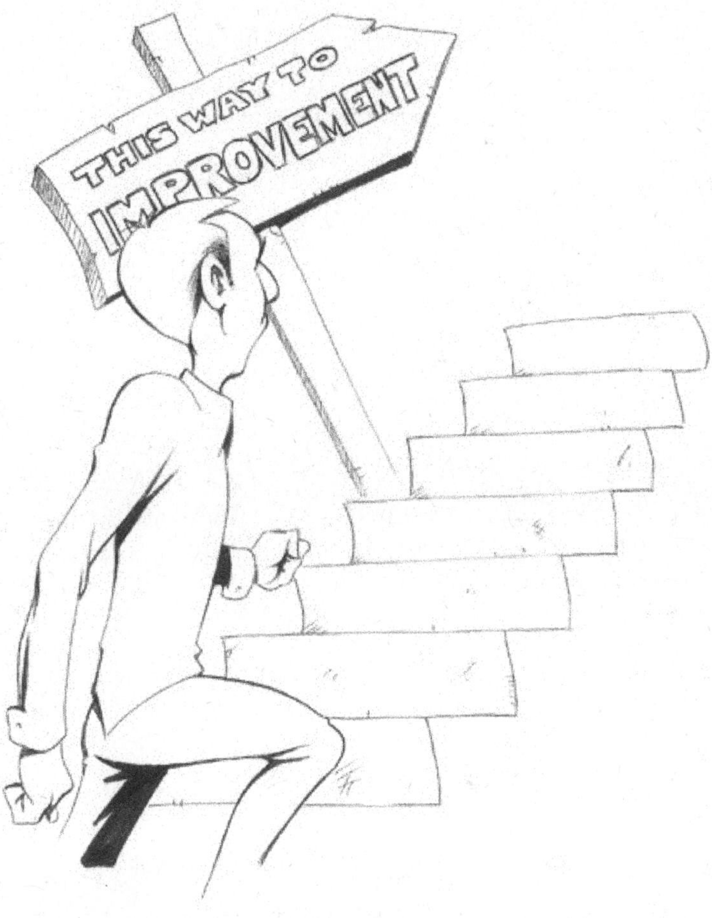

overcoming
functional neurological symptoms:
A Five Areas Approach

SECTION 1: Introduction

A diagnosis of functional neurological symptoms is much more common than you might think. Research in four major neurological centres suggests that about one in three people attending neurology outpatient clinics have this diagnosis.

What are functional neurological symptoms?

The diagnosis of functional neurological symptoms covers a wide range of difficulties in how your body works. These include:

Paralysis or weakness of an arm or leg	Pain in your arms, legs or joints (knees, hips, etc.)
Double or blurred vision	Chest pain
Partial or total loss of vision	Feeling your heart pound or race
Partial or total loss of hearing	Problems with your memory or concentration
Difficulty swallowing or a lump in the throat	Shortness of breath
Difficulty speaking or slurred speech	Stomach pain
Lack of co-ordination or balance	Constipation, loose bowels or diarrhoea
Seizure or fit	Nausea, gas or indigestion
An anxiety attack (suddenly feeling fear or panic)	Feeling tired or having low energy
Shaking or tremor	Trouble sleeping
Headaches	Little interest or pleasure in doing things
Dizziness	Feeling down, depressed or hopeless
Fainting spells	'Nerves' or feeling anxious or on edge
Loss of sensation, numbness or tingling	Worrying about a lot of different things
Back pain	Having flashbacks to stressful events

Functional neurological symptoms can affect anybody no matter how old, what gender or race. It affects people from all parts of society. It doesn't matter whether you are working, retired, a student or unemployed – anyone can develop this problem. Half of those people with these symptoms are still working.

How is the diagnosis of functional neurological symptoms made?

Your neurologist will make the diagnosis based on two key factors:

- Your *clinical history* (what you tell them) – how your symptoms have developed and how they affect you.
- Your *physical examination*: especially an expert neurological examination.

Sometimes, based on your assessment, specialist investigations may be recommended. You can find out more about these in Workbook 2. Please note that these investigations may well have been previously completed by your GP.

> KEY POINT
> **The diagnosis of functional neurological symptoms can be made as accurately as any other diagnosis. The diagnosis usually means that further tests are not required. The treatment package described in these workbooks is designed to help you overcome your symptoms.**

The overcoming functional neurological symptoms treatment package

This first workbook contains an overview of the treatment approaches people can use to help overcome problems caused by functional neurological symptoms. It covers:

- How to use the workbook.
- The diagnosis of functional neurological symptoms.
- Understanding the impact of these symptoms by looking at the effect **on five key areas** of your life. These are:
  - Your physical symptoms/feelings in your body
  - Your thoughts
  - Your feelings or emotions
  - The impact of all these on your activity levels and life
  - The situations, relationship and practical problems you face.
- How to use this approach to improve things. By using the different workbooks in the course you can slowly put things back to normal in your life.
- A brief description of the workbooks that make up the rest of this course. This will help you to choose which workbooks will be most helpful for you.

You can use the workbooks by yourself or with your healthcare practitioner. You may find that it is also helpful going through them with a friend or family member (see Practical toolbox E – Illness, symptoms and other people).

KEY POINT

Many people notice that they feel slightly worse to begin with as they use this approach. This is usually only temporary and is an important part of the process of recovery.

How to use the workbooks

We recommend that any workbook you use is completed over a period of a week or two. Completing the entire course of workbooks is therefore likely to take more than a month. But putting the techniques into practice might take longer than you think. It does take an investment of your time for these approaches to work.

- ★ There is a lot of information in each workbook, so the workbooks are divided into clear sections covering each topic.
- ★ You might find it helpful to read one section at a time.
- ★ Try to **answer all the questions** asked. The process of having to **stop, think and reflect** on how the questions might be relevant to you is an important part of getting better.
- ★ You will probably find that some aspects of each workbook are more useful to you at the moment than others. **Write down** your own notes of key points in the margins or in the *My notes* area at the back of the workbook to help you remember information that has been helpful. Plan to **review** your notes regularly to help you apply what you have learned.
- ★ Once you have read through an entire workbook once, **put it to one side** and then **re-read it** again a few days later. It may be that different parts of it become clearer, or seem more useful on second reading.
- ★ Within each workbook, important areas are labelled as **key points**. Certain areas that are covered may not be relevant for everyone. Such areas will be clearly identified so that you can choose to skip optional material if you wish.

> KEY POINT
> **There is no right or wrong way to use this manual. Some people like to fill in a lot of detail but others prefer brief notes. Do whatever you feel helps you reflect on your situation. The information you record is simply to help you.**

Every person has a different experience. In the workbooks we will use some specific examples but some will seem more relevant to you than others. The object of the workbooks is to allow your own experience to form the basis for treatment.

When times are difficult ...

Functional neurological symptoms can make life seem like a real struggle. This is why choosing to commit yourself to the approach is important, and why we recommend using the workbooks together with someone else who can encourage and support you. Taking small steps can make a really big difference to how you feel.

> KEY POINT
> **Adjusting just a few small things in your life can result in big benefits.**

How the workbook will help you

Symptoms have an effect on **every** aspect of your life. Think about the experience of having flu. The flu virus causes symptoms such as a runny nose, temperature and aching muscles. But it also affects other key parts of our lives. You can have:

- *Altered thinking*: you may not think as clearly as usual and may find it difficult to make decisions.
- *Altered feelings*: you may not enjoy things as much as usual – and not feel very cheerful.
- *Altered behaviour*: you may have to go to bed, take medicines such as throat lozenges and paracetamol, and rest. You may not feel like going about your usual life activities such as meeting friends or going out.
- Symptoms that also have *an impact on those around you*. For example, others may make your meals and bring you drinks. If there is no one around to do these things, people might feel increasingly isolated.

In flu, these symptoms resolve over a week or so. What happens when symptoms last for far longer than this or are more severe?

Illness doesn't just affect our physical health. It affects our work, family, social life and hobbies, and all our relationships. This can sometimes feel like having a mountain to climb. You might feel that your symptoms have taken over your life and you'll never be yourself again.

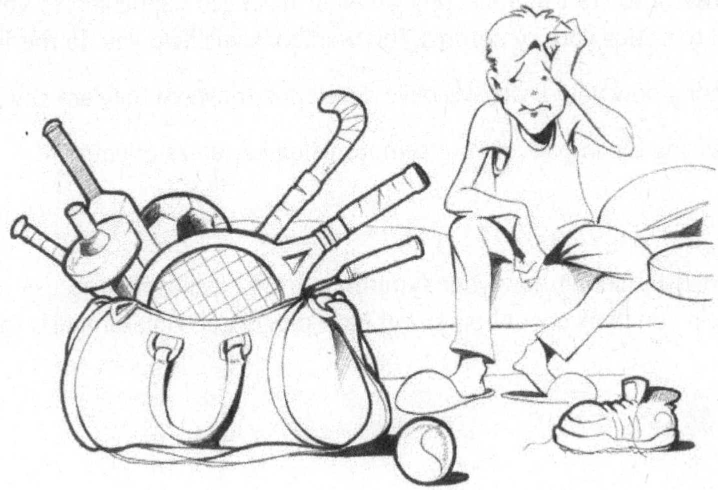

The workbooks all use an approach to help you work out how your problems are affecting you in different areas of your life. This treatment approach is based on a cognitive behavioural therapy (CBT or talking therapy) approach. This therapy can help people cope with a wide range of health problems such as heart disease, diabetes, cancer, tiredness, pain and anxiety. It teaches you skills to cope with your symptoms.

SECTION 2: Starting your own self-assessment

It can be useful to start by reflecting on what has been happening to you since you first began to notice your symptoms. This workbook will help you do this in two ways:

1 Considering how your problems have developed to where they are now.

2 Summarising the impact of your symptoms on key areas of your life.

How my symptoms have developed

One way of considering how your symptoms have developed is to use a **time line**. This can help you think about how things have progressed. An example is shown below.

Example time line

★ Beginning

Paul (age 35), works as a civil servant.

July 2002. Car accident

October 2002. Started getting bad headaches

Next 6 months tried on lots of medications by my GP

May 2003. Started to get tingling in my right hand

Summer 2003. On holiday, felt right leg give way

Had medical tests while on holiday

Autumn/Winter 2003. Tingling comes and goes

January 2004. Wife gives birth to our daughter

March 2004. Right hand very weak and sometimes 'won't work'

My GP suggests referral to neurology

May 2004. Sick leave from work because of pain tingling and occasional paralysis

October 2004. Seen by neurologist, no specific disease found

★ Today

Told by neurologist I have a functional disorder

Task

Write in your own time line of the progress of your current problem in the space below. Give a general overview of key changes that have happened since the symptoms became a major problem for you.

Time line

Beginning (a time when I last was well)

Today

The Five Areas assessment

We already know from our own experiences that health problems are very complex and affect us in many ways. A *Five Areas assessment* will provide you with a clear summary of the difficulties you are facing in each of the following areas:

1 Symptoms/feelings in your body.

2 Altered thinking.

3 Altered feelings (also called moods or emotions).

4 Altered behaviour or activity levels (with reduced activity, avoidance or unhelpful behaviours).

5 Your life situation, relationships, practical problems (i.e. the people and events around you).

Below is an example of how Mary, who has a common illness, responds to being unwell and the impact it has on all five aspects of her life.

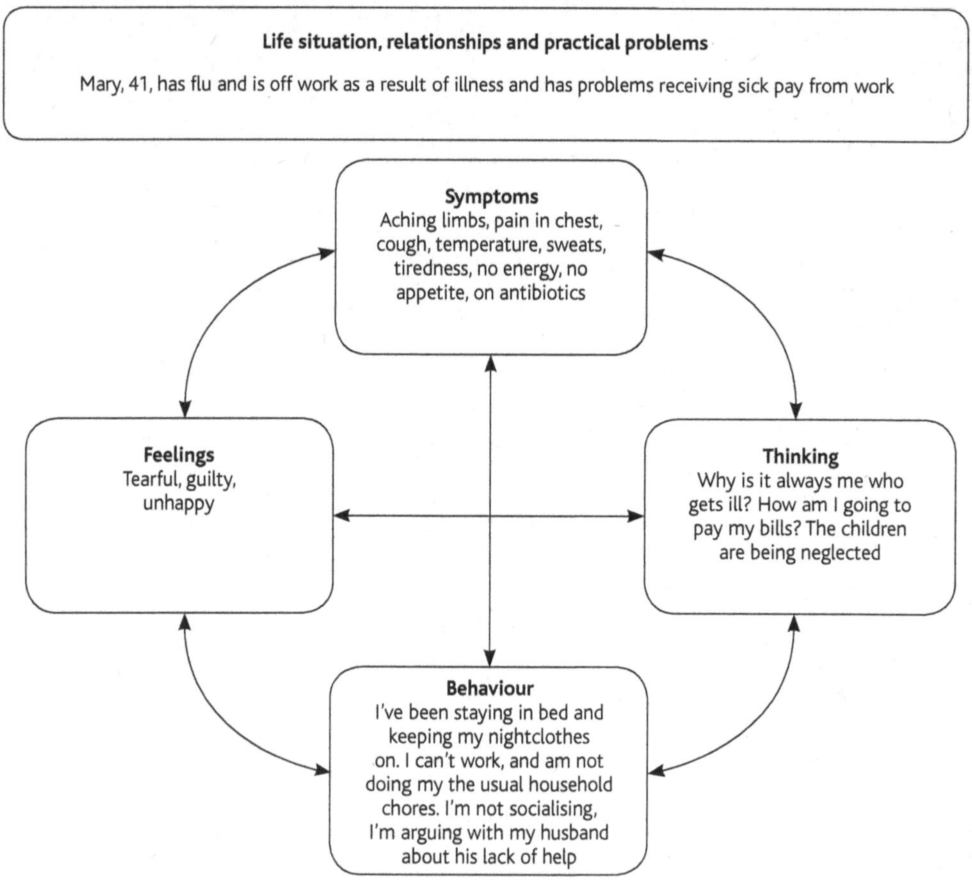

The Five Areas assessment model of Mary.

Look at the arrows in the diagram. Each of these five areas affects each other and offers possible areas of change to improve how Mary feels. Because of the links between the areas, the physical impact of Mary's illness influences many other important aspects of her life. It also shows how much illness can affect people. For example, being ill can have emotional consequences. This is especially the case where symptoms stop you living your life as you would wish, or when illness lasts for many months or years. Living with uncertainty, and with long-term illness, can grind people down.

Mary's example shows how much even a short-term (sometimes called 'acute') illness and very common problem with health can affect people. **How you think about your illness can also play an important part**. The Five Areas assessment shows that what a person thinks about a situation or problem may affect how they feel emotionally and physically, and also alters what they do. Finally, other important things going on in your life – such as relationships, jobs (or lack of a job) – can all affect how you are.

Don't worry if this approach seems hard to understand at first. In the next section of the workbook you'll have the chance to complete your own Five Areas assessment. This will make the approach clearer to you.

SECTION 3: Carrying out your own Five Areas assessment

A **Five Areas assessment** can be helpful in understanding how your symptoms are affecting you.

> **REMINDER**
> The five areas are: symptoms; thinking; feelings/emotions/mood; behaviour or activity levels in the face of illness; and your situation, relationship or practical problems. Think about how your health problems have affected you in the past few weeks.

Area 1: Symptoms

An important point to think about with functional neurological symptoms is the symptoms themselves.

Listing your symptoms

Symptom	*First started*	*How often do you have it?*	*What helps?*	*What makes it worse?*
Fatigue	*December 2009*	*Every day*	*Resting*	*Exercise or activity*

Physical symptoms can be made worse by uncertainty, frustration, stress or demoralisation. For example, when you feel tense, you might also notice feeling restless and unable to relax. Feelings of mental tension can also cause physical tension in our muscles and joints. This may cause shakiness, pain, weakness or tiredness.

It can be surprising how tiring stress can be. Some people may feel completely exhausted when they have felt stressed for a time. Their muscles are so tense it can seem as if they have run a marathon all day. This muscle tension can cause other problems, such as tension headaches, or stomach or chest pains. Anxiety can also cause other physical symptoms. A feeling of being hot or cold, sweaty or clammy is common. Your heart may seem to be racing, and you may feel fuzzy-headed or disconnected from things.

Low mood or depression can also lead to a number of symptoms.

Symptoms that can be worsened by stress or low mood	*Tick here if you notice this symptom*
Pain – especially pain that is worse in the mornings, and which is unaffected by painkillers. Examples are tension headaches, stomach pain, eyestrain or chest pain	☐
Muscle tension/shakiness	☐
Tiredness and low energy	☐
Reduced or increased appetite (comfort eating)	☐
Weight loss or gain (as a result of comfort eating and under-activity)	☐
Reduced concentration – can't keep focused	☐
Problems going off or staying asleep. You may wake up earlier than normal, feeling unrested and not be able to get off to sleep again	☐
Feeling dizzy/fuzzy-headed or cut off from things	☐
There may be anxiety about sex and avoidance of sex as a result. Loss of sex drive	☐
Butterflies, loose bowels, sickness, churning stomach, going to the toilet frequently	☐
Restless and tense. Rapid heart/palpitations. Sweaty, clammy, shaky	☐
Dry mouth. Shallow rapid breathing	☐
Constipation	☐

Summary for Area 1: Symptoms

Having read about this area:

Q Overall, do you think these symptoms affect you? Yes ☐ No ☐

You will find out more about symptoms in Workbook 2.

Area 2: Thinking

When facing symptoms, people can often feel overwhelmed and uncertain about the future. You may not realise your strengths and ability to cope with your symptoms. Things can seem to be out of control.

How do you respond when you notice worrying thoughts about illness?

A common response from people around us when trying to cope with health problems is to say: 'Try not to think about it.'

Experiment

To see if trying not to think about worrying thoughts about illness is effective, do this practical experiment. Try very hard for the next 30 seconds not to think about a white polar bear.

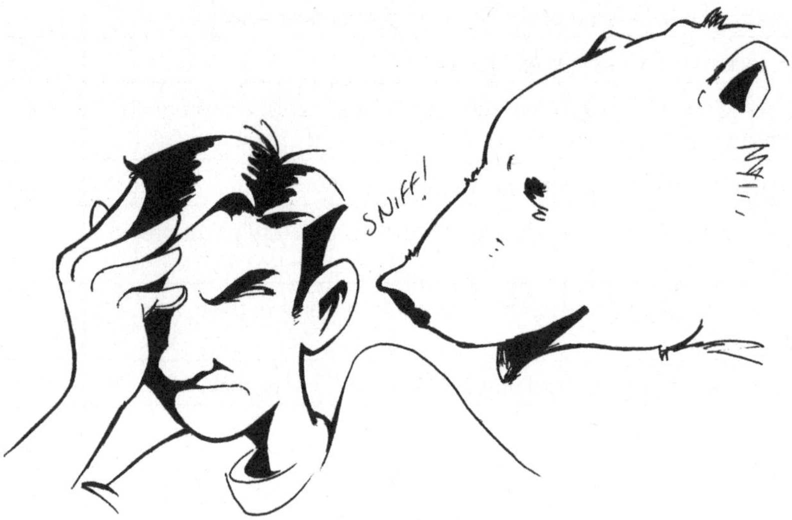

After you have done this, think about what happened. Was it easy not to think about the polar bear, or did it take a lot of effort?

You may have noticed that trying hard not to think about the bear actually made it worse. Alternatively, you may have spent a lot of mental effort trying hard to think about something else such as a black polar bear? For many people, trying hard to ignore their worrying thoughts doesn't work and may actually worsen the problem.

Q Do I end up putting a lot of mental effort into trying hard not to think worrying thoughts? Yes ☐ No ☐

Q If I try not to think the thoughts, does it work? Yes ☐ No ☐

You will learn about *unhelpful thinking styles* that can affect anyone from time to time. During times of distress, especially when someone is struggling hard against their symptoms, they become more frequent and are harder to dismiss. Focusing on problems means they can often build up in your mind without actually being tackled. People may see their symptoms in catastrophic ways and predict that the very worst will occur.

However, such thinking styles can be unrealistic, extreme and unhelpful. When such thoughts dominate your thinking, they can make you feel worse.

Why are such thoughts so unhelpful?

The unhelpful thoughts can worsen how you feel emotionally and physically. This then can unhelpfully alter what you do in both the short and the longer term.

Unhelpful thinking causes

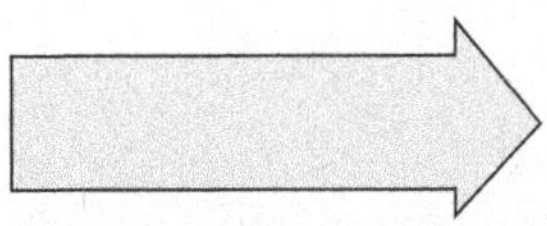

Unhelpful mood changes

You may feel more down, guilty, upset, anxious ashamed, stressed or angry

Unhelpful behaviour changes

You may stop or reduce what you normally do, or start to avoid things that worry you or cause stress. Conversely, you may start to act in ways that seem to help but which end up backfiring and worsen how you feel in the longer term

Images and mental pictures – an important part of how people think

Some people notice *mental pictures or images* in their mind when they think about their illness. The images may be moving or still, or be in black and white or in colour. They may include mental pictures of painful parts of the body such as joints, or pictures of a brain tumour, multiple sclerosis or being in a wheelchair or alone. As with all thoughts, mental images can be inaccurate or **portray the very worst** outcome. They may sometimes worry about scary things happening and feel even more anxious or upset as a result.

Do you think you are prone to noticing intrusive, upsetting thoughts or mental pictures? Yes ☐ No ☐

Write down any upsetting thoughts or mental images here. If it is a mental image you may wish to draw it or describe it in writing.

Summary for Area 2: Thinking

Having read about this area:

Overall, do you experience unhelpful thinking? (actual thoughts or images) Yes ☐ No ☐

These problems are potential areas for change. You will find out more about the steps to take to tackle these problems in Workbook 5.

Area 3: Feelings

Emotional reactions to illness vary. This is because it depends on whether you see your symptoms as overwhelming, frustrating, demoralising or just a nuisance.

> KEY POINT
>
> **When someone has symptoms, they often feel emotional. This is true of cancer, chest and heart problems, as well as functional neurological symptoms.**

Everyone reacts differently when it comes to emotions. Some of us just switch off and don't notice anything – no matter how unsettling the symptoms might appear to others. Some of us just don't want to think about what is going on ('denial') and see 'just getting on with things' as important. Some of us find an inner calm or peace through a personal religious faith or philosophy. However, the majority of people have a variety of emotional reactions from time to time.

For example:

- *Frustration* and *demoralisation* can sometimes *grind people down* so that they wish to withdraw from treatment, and feel low or depressed.
- Feelings of *tension* can cause symptoms of *physical pain*, and result in changes to breathing and heart rate.
- You may find yourself becoming *angry* at the symptoms, or at doctors or relatives who don't seem to understand.
- Others may try to avoid talking about the symptoms, and try to hide the problem as a result of strong feelings of *embarrassment*.
- *Anxious fears* about illness can make people feel scared of doing things. You may *start to avoid* specific situations, people or places that you believe worsen how you feel. The result can be an *undermining of confidence* and an *increasingly restricted life*.
- Sometimes anxious fears can lead to *anxious checking*. Going from one healthcare practitioner or source of information to another means people may never really give any approach a chance to lead to improvement. They may become confused by all sorts of conflicting ideas, investigations and treatments.

It's important to remember that these different emotional responses are all normal and understandable. They are important both because this **is** how you may feel and because sometimes these emotions can themselves add to problems.

KEY POINT

Emotional reactions are a part of how people react and cope with functional neurological symptoms. They are not a sign of weakness or of failing to cope. They are an important part of a person – and of your response to illness.

Use this box to note down anything you have noticed about yourself and your feelings or emotions.

Summary for Area 3: Feelings/emotions

Having read about this area:

Overall, do you have altered feelings? Yes ☐ No ☐

These problems are potential targets for change. You will find out more about the steps to take to tackle these by reading the other workbooks in the course.

Area 4: Behaviour

Being ill can lead to changes in behaviour and activity levels. For example, it is a common reaction to *reduce what you do* in order to rest and recover. You may also start to *avoid doing things* that seem just too much or too difficult. You may also try to respond by altering what you do to improve how you feel. Later in this workbook, and in Workbooks 3 and 4, you'll see that this *altered behaviour* can sometimes be a helpful part of recovery. But sometimes it can backfire and become part of the problem (an *unhelpful behaviour*).

Altered behaviour (i): reduced activity

When someone feels ill it is normal to find it is difficult doing things. This is because of:

- Feeling ill.
- Low energy and tiredness ('I'm too ill/tired'). Or physical problems such as stiffness or weakness.
- Low mood and little sense of enjoyment or achievement when things are done.
- Negative thinking and reduced enthusiasm to do things ('I just can't be bothered').

The consequence is that things you used to do before that previously gave you a sense of pleasure or achievement may be squeezed out of your life. A **vicious circle of reduced activity** may result.

You can find out more about this vicious circle and the effects of reduced activity in Workbooks 3 and 4.

Altered behaviour (ii): avoidance

Anxiety can sometimes be understandably present as part of the reaction to illness. You may have worries or concerns about the illness itself, your ability to cope, the reactions of others, and what will happen in the future. Anxiety of any sort causes people to avoid situations that may seem threatening. This can include *situations* that either make you more anxious, or make you feel physically worse. You may find yourself avoiding different situations, objects, people or places because of how you feel. A **vicious circle of avoidance** can result. The impact is often an increasingly restricted lifestyle, undermined confidence and additional distress.

Example

Someone with anxious fears after having a heart attack will avoid any situations or activities that they think might put them 'at risk'. They may therefore avoid exercise or other usual activities.

You can learn more about this in Workbook 4.

Altered behaviour (iii): unhelpful behaviours

One problem is that everyone has expectations of how they 'should', 'must', 'ought' to react when they are sick. We *should* stop doing things. We *must* seek treatment and take this. We *ought to* get better and move on from our illness to recovery. We *should* act differently when ill – wear different clothes, eat different foods, rest, look and act ill. These 'rules' often work well for short-term illnesses such as colds, flu, a broken ankle. They also work for problems such as appendicitis, which have a clear cause and also resolve over a number of days and weeks. It can be so much more difficult if symptoms are unexpected and are quite scary, or if they last for a long time.

When you become unwell, you may respond by changing what you do in a number of different ways. Sometimes these changes can be *helpful* – for example seeing a doctor or other healthcare practitioner. Sometimes, however, they can become unhelpful and worsen how you feel. For example, pushing yourself too hard and then feeling worse. Although this can make you feel better in the short term, in the longer term it may unhelpfully affect you physically, emotionally and in your relationships. A **vicious circle of unhelpful behaviour** can occur. Remember that although often unhelpful behaviours make you feel better in the short term, in the longer term they backfire and add to your problems.

A useful question to identify your unhelpful behaviours is to ask 'What am I doing differently to cope with how I feel?'. Checklists for this can be found in Workbook 4 and will help you to identify any unhelpful behaviour in your life.

KEY POINT

Remember that the reason why people reduce activity, avoid things or start an unhelpful behaviour is to feel better – at least in the short term. Although they lead to a short-term relief in symptoms, this doesn't last. Any symptoms or anxiety/stress usually quickly returns to the same or an even higher level.

Summary for Area 4: Behaviour (reduced activity, avoidance or unhelpful behaviours)

Having read about this area:

Overall, do you have altered behaviour? Yes ☐ No ☐

These difficulties are potential targets for change. You will find out more about what steps to take to tackle these in Workbooks 3 and 4.

Area 5: Situation, relationship and practical problems

Practical problems or difficulties in relationships are common. When people face several problems at the same time, they may begin to feel overwhelmed. This may be worse when you feel ill. Health problems can reduce your ability to respond well to other problems. You may struggle with everyday tasks such as housework. These everyday difficulties are just one more source of unwanted pressure. Symptoms often seem worse when several life pressures occur at the same time. So these practical problems and life difficulties may include:

- Debts, housing or other problems.
- Problems in relationships with family, friends or colleagues, etc. Having an illness can sometimes affect relationships – and those around you may not know how best to help.
- Other difficult situations that you face such as problems at home or work (or lack of work, for example unemployment or problems with benefits).

Use this box to note down anything you have noticed about yourself in relation to your situation, relationships or practical problems.

Summary for Area 5: Situation, relationship and practical problems

Having read about this area:

Overall, do you have problems in this area? Yes ☐ No ☐

These problems are potential targets for change. You will find out more about the steps to take to tackle these in Workbook 3 and the Toolbox.

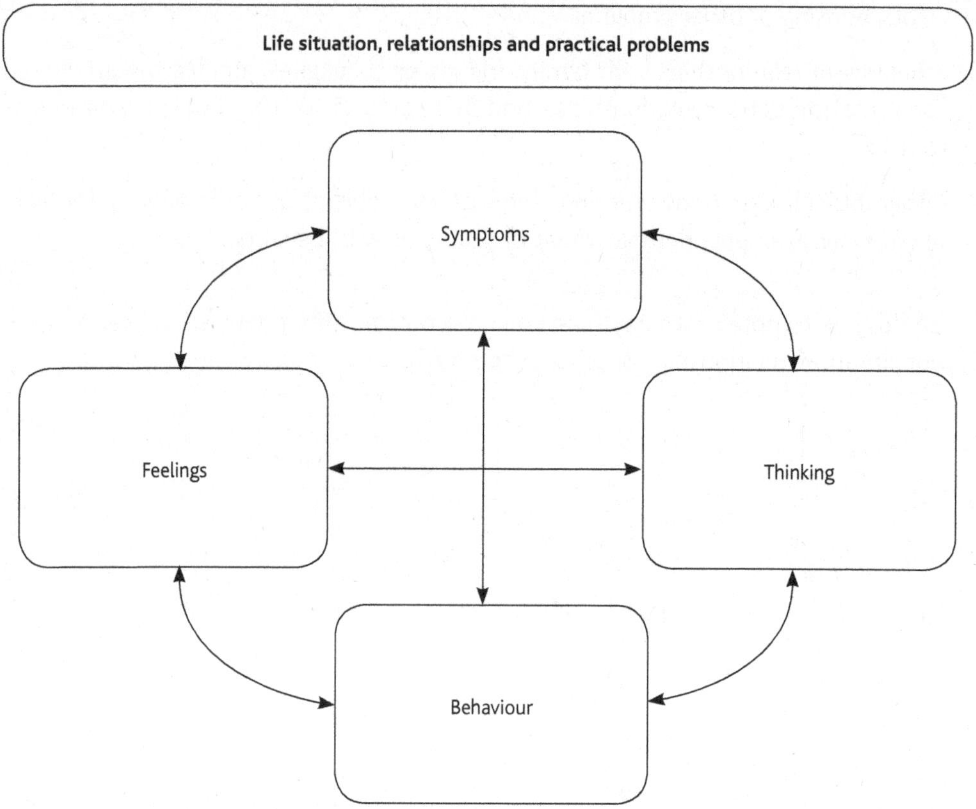

The Five Areas model.

You have now learnt about each of the five areas. Before you move on, think about what you have learned. How does what you have read help you to make sense of your symptoms?

The purpose of the Five Areas assessment is to help you plan the areas you need to focus on to bring about change. The workbooks in this course can help you begin to tackle each of the five problem areas.

SECTION 4: Next steps

Some people find it's helpful to discuss what they have learned with someone who knows them well, such as a partner, close friend or family member. People around you might have noticed things, which you have not, and it also might help them to understand just how much your current situation affects every aspect of your life.

The main problem areas seen in functional neurological symptoms are the:

- Symptoms.
- Altered thinking (with extreme and unhelpful thinking).
- Altered feelings/mood/emotions.
- Altered behaviour (with reduced activity, avoidance or unhelpful behaviours).
- Current situations, relationship or practical problems.

You will have now thought about each of these five areas and how they might apply to you. Links can occur between any of the areas. Because of this, aiming to alter **any** of the areas can help.

> KEY POINT
>
> **By defining your problems, you have now identified possible target areas to focus on. The key is to make sure that you do things one step at a time. Slow, steady steps are more likely to result in improvement, rather than starting very enthusiastically and then running out of steam.**

Short-, medium- and longer-term goals

You are more likely to get better if you have a clear plan and stick to it. This means choosing a specific target to start with and leaving other areas for the time being. Setting yourself targets will help you to focus on how to make the changes needed to get better.

To do this you will need to decide:

Long-term targets: where you want to be in six months or a year

Medium-term targets: changes to be put in place over the next few weeks

Short-term targets: changes you can make today, tomorrow and next week

Use the table below to help you decide which workbooks to read first and over the next few weeks and months.

	Tick when completed		
	Short-term goals (plan to read in the next week or so)	*Medium-term goals (plan to read over the next few weeks)*	*Long-term goals (plan to read over the next few months)*
Workbook 1: Introduction	✓		
Workbook 2: Your brain and body, and how these link to symptoms			
Workbook 3: A Five Areas Approach to rehabilitation			
Workbook 4: Behaviours			
Workbook 5: Noticing and changing unhelpful thinking			
Toolbox A: Overcoming reduced activity and avoidance			
Toolbox B: Practical problem solving			
Toolbox C: How to become more assertive			
Toolbox D: Healthy living			
Toolbox E: Illness, symptoms and other people			

KEY POINT

In order to change, you will need to choose to apply what you will learn regularly throughout the week, and not just when you read the workbook. The workbooks will encourage you to do this by sometimes suggesting certain tasks or experiments for you to carry out. These tasks will:

- **Help you to put into practice what you have learned.**
- **Gather information so that you can get the most out of it.**

SECTION 5: Summary

In this workbook you have learned:

- **How to use this workbook.**
- **How people respond to symptoms.**
- **The key ways that symptoms can affect your life.**
- **The Five Areas assessment: the symptoms, thinking, emotional changes and behaviour that make up your response to the challenge of illness, as well as the situations, relationship and practical problems you face.**
- **The areas you need to tackle in order to overcome your own problems.**

Putting into practice what you have learned

- Choose **two episodes** over the next week when you feel either more physically ill or distressed. Use the blank Five Areas assessment that follows this section to record the impact on your body, thinking, mood and behaviour at that time. Try to write a summary of how you feel in each of the five areas. What impact did your symptoms have on how you thought and felt and what you did during these two episodes? Can you identify any examples of reduced activity, avoidance or unhelpful behaviours? You will find a blank example, with helpful questions, on page 30. You can photocopy or draw additional copies of the diagram as you need it, and keep the sheet handy. You can also download copies from www.fiveareas.com.

- Identify your current goal – it may be to move on to the next workbook or to re-read this one.

My current goal

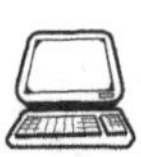

You can get additional help and support in problem solving at www.livinglifetothefull.com

Acknowledgements

The use of the Five Areas assessment model and associated language is used from the Overcoming Five Areas series by permission of Hodder Arnold Publishers and Dr C Williams. Illustrations are by Keith Chan and are reproduced with permission.

A request for feedback

An important factor in the development of all the Five Areas assessment workbooks is that the content is updated on a regular basis based on feedback from users and practitioners. If there are areas within any of the workbooks that you find hard to understand, or seem poorly written, please let us know and we will try to improve things in future. We are sorry that we are unable to provide any specific replies or advice on treatment.

To provide feedback, please contact us via:

Email: feedback@fiveareas.com

Mail: Dr Chris Williams, Five Areas, PO Box 9, Drymen, G63 0HA.

My notes

A Five Areas assessment of a specific time when I feel worse

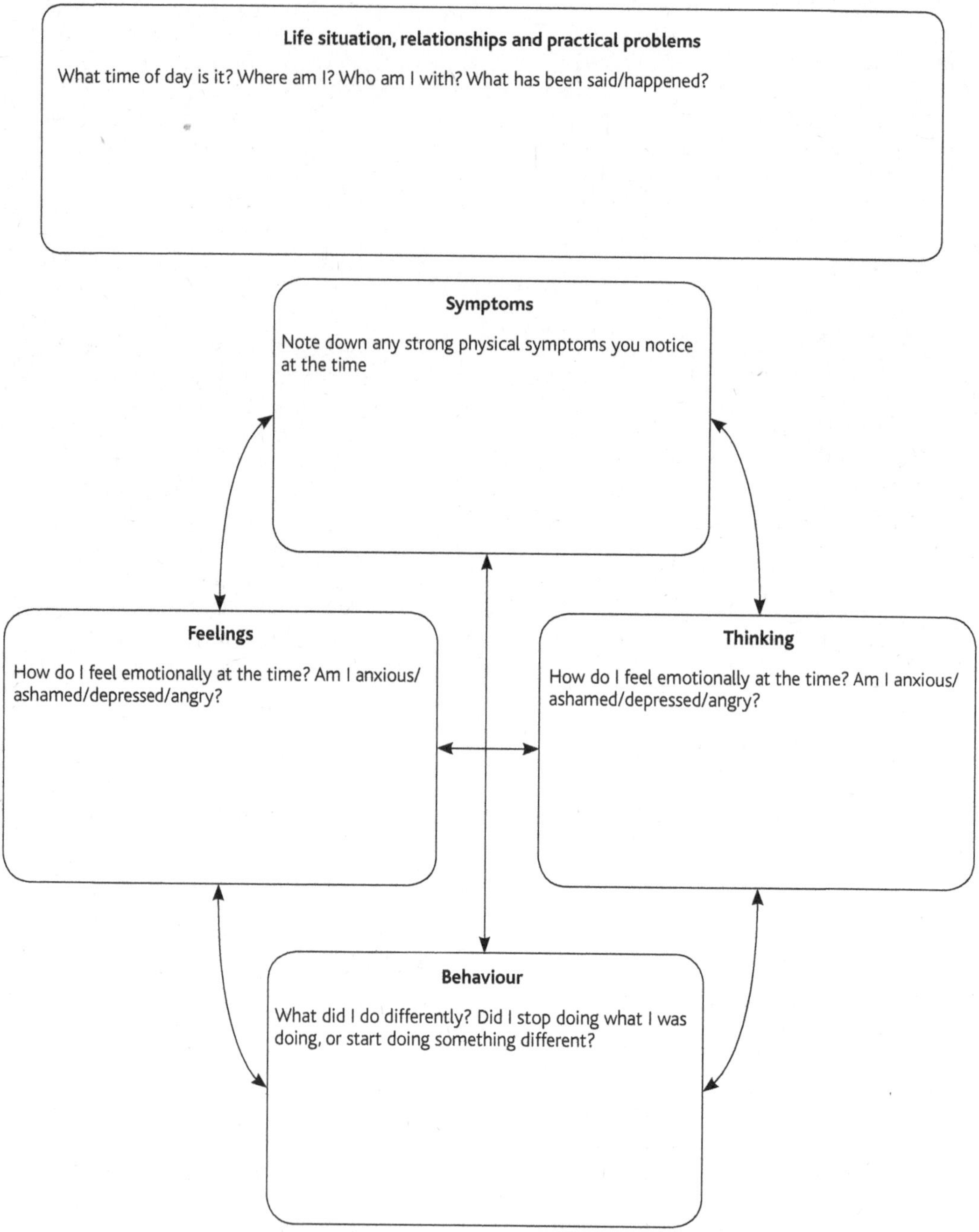

Workbook 2

Your brain and body, and how these link to symptoms

overcoming
functional neurological symptoms:
A Five Areas Approach

INTRODUCTION

The aim of this workbook is to look at your symptoms in more detail and to help you understand more about how your body works.

This workbook will cover:

- **Common neurological symptoms.**
- **How doctors make diagnoses.**
- **How your brain and body works.**
- **Uncertainty.**
- **Medicine and other treatments.**

SECTION 1: Common neurological symptoms

Before we look in more detail at your own symptoms, let's take a look at two examples.

Example: Naz's story

A year ago Naz noticed he had more headaches than usual. Soon they were coming every day. At work he was under a lot of pressure. A colleague was off sick and Naz had to cover some of her work too. There were deadlines coming up and he knew his boss was keen to meet them. There were rumours of redundancies across the company. Naz also spent a lot of his spare time helping his parents as his father had had a stroke the previous summer. Naz would often visit them in the evenings and take them out in the car for a drive once a week.

Naz was worried about his headaches but thought they were due to stress. He took painkillers and tried to carry on as normal.

One Wednesday at work Naz collapsed. His colleagues rushed to help him and someone called an ambulance. Naz could barely stand. His legs felt like they were made of jelly and he was tingling down his right side. He found it difficult to talk and was very scared that he might be having a stroke like his father. The ambulance arrived and he was given oxygen. He was taken to the accident and emergency department (A&E) where a nurse took some blood and attached a monitor to him. While he lay waiting for the doctor, Naz's symptoms got better. By the time the doctor came all that was left was a headache. The doctor did not seem to mind and spent quite a bit of time checking him over. He told Naz that he could find nothing wrong and that he should visit his GP, who could look into it a little further.

Naz went back to work the next day and his colleagues were very surprised to see him. He found it difficult to explain what had happened and was embarrassed at their questions.

Later that morning, he noticed that his right leg was shaking under the desk and when he tried to get up he felt very unsteady. He began to feel more unwell and decided to go home early. He tried not to make a fuss. On his way out he was holding onto the railings in case he fell. He felt that he was tilting to the right. His leg felt very weak. He caught a taxi to his GP's surgery. The GP saw him quickly and examined him thoroughly but could not find anything wrong. Naz's symptoms again wore off. His GP arranged for him to be seen at the local neurology department and to have a brain scan. She warned him there might be some wait for his appointments but she was fairly sure that there was nothing seriously wrong. Over the next few weeks Naz's symptoms came and went. His leg seemed to be getting weaker and often gave way under him. He continued to have headaches.

He bought himself a blood pressure monitor and used it quite often through the day. He was reluctant to go out as he worried he would fall or collapse. He stopped going to his regular football game. He wondered whether stress could cause a stroke. He felt guilty that he could not help his parents and asked his sister to take over for a while. Even though his GP had been quite reassuring, he was still worried about what was happening and hoped he would get his hospital appointments soon.

As you can see, Naz was having a number of common neurological symptoms. Naturally he was worried he might have something very seriously wrong. After reading his story, you may be surprised to find when he eventually saw the neurologist and had his scan there was no evidence of serious illness. The diagnosis was functional neurological symptoms.

Kate also has neurological symptoms. Her story is told below.

Example: Kate's story

Kate has had seizures for two years. When the fits first started they were unpredictable and came out of the blue. She would collapse to the floor and feel quite 'out of it' when she came round. She was not sure whether she was unconscious for long and had difficulty remembering what had happened. People told her she jerked and shook sometimes. She found it difficult to look after her three teenage children, and her mother had to help out. She often had seizures at work and would end up being sent home. Before this Kate had always been healthy. She had had occasional stomach problems in the past (stomach acid coming up into her mouth) and was still bothered by this at times but medication had helped.

When the seizures started, Kate often saw her doctor and occasionally ended up in A&E. All her tests were normal and her doctor thought that they should wait and see what happened. She was given some diazepam in case she needed it and this helped at times. Her doctor was reassuring but Kate was still worried.

Kate's best friend had epilepsy and she had seen her having fits. Kate was able to tell her friends and family how to look after her and gradually she returned to a more normal life. Her children stopped phoning her relatives when she had a fit at home. Instead they would take over making their tea or whatever she was doing. Her work colleagues allowed her to cut back some of her duties and she was able to leave early if she felt a fit coming on. Not everyone was so sympathetic and her sister even told her she was faking it. This upset Kate very much.

Over time she was able to predict days when she might have a fit. She also noticed other symptoms that accompanied her seizures. That is, the seizures seemed to come if she was tired, felt under stress, had drunk wine or coffee or had eaten certain foods. Sometimes she had a headache across the back of her head and felt dizzy before her fit. Her hands tingled, she felt vague and had difficulty finding her words. She often felt as if she was cut off from the rest of the world. This was a weird feeling which she found difficult to describe to her family. She noticed that when her stomach was playing up she was much more likely to have a seizure. She wondered if different foods might be the cause. Her doctor thought that this was unlikely though and sometimes Kate felt disbelieved by him too.

Over time Kate became frustrated with her doctor, as no one could tell her exactly what was wrong. She asked for a second opinion and was referred to the local neurology department. When the neurologist saw Kate, she was given a diagnosis of non-epileptic seizures and told there was a good chance she would get better. Kate was very relieved to finally be told what was wrong with her. She also found her symptoms easier to explain to the people around her.

This is another example of a functional neurological disorder. You might feel there are some similarities between your own story and those of Naz and Kate. You may even share some of their symptoms. While no two people are exactly the same, such symptoms are very familiar to neurologists. Often there is a mixture of symptoms. They can be disabling and cause distress and affect how you live your life day to day. You might also recognise some of the worries and frustrations that Naz and Kate experienced.

Your symptoms

In Workbook 1 you filled out a time line of your own symptoms. It might be helpful now to use the checklist below to describe these in more detail.

Checklist of symptoms

Paralysis or weakness of an arm or leg	☐
Double or blurred vision	☐
Partial or total loss of vision	☐
Partial or total loss of hearing	☐
Difficulty swallowing or a lump in the throat	☐

Difficulty speaking or slurred speech	☐
Lack of co-ordination or balance	☐
Seizure or fit	☐
An anxiety attack (suddenly feeling fear or panic)	☐
Shaking or tremor	☐
Headaches	☐
Dizziness	☐
Fainting spells	☐
Loss of sensation, numbness or tingling	☐
Back pain	☐
Pain in your arms, legs or joints (knees, hips, etc.)	☐
Chest pain	☐
Feeling your heart pound or race	☐
Problems with your memory or concentration	☐
Shortness of breath	☐
Stomach pain	☐
Constipation, loose bowels or diarrhoea	☐
Nausea, gas or indigestion	☐
Feeling tired or having low energy	☐
Trouble sleeping	☐
Little interest or pleasure in doing things	☐
Feeling down, depressed or hopeless	☐
'Nerves' or feeling anxious or on edge	☐
Worrying about a lot of different things	☐
Having flashbacks to stressful events	☐

It seems a very large list but of course not everyone will have all the symptoms listed here and you may only notice one or two of them. Or you may find you have several.

It can be difficult to imagine how all of these symptoms might be caused by one diagnosis. Often people are puzzled how the neurologist has made their diagnosis.

The following sections explain how doctors make their decisions and how the human body works.

SECTION 2: How doctors make diagnoses

When a person become unwell, changes happen to the body. Sometimes they are sudden, and at other times they are more gradual. You might go to your doctor to get help. You will want to know:

- What is it? (*Diagnosis*)
- What caused it? (*Aetiology*)
- What can you, or others, do about it? (*Treatment*)
- What will happen? (*Prognosis*)

Your doctor will try to answer all these questions. Sometimes it is not made clear how doctors make their decisions. This can leave people a little bewildered and unsure.

What happens first?

When you go to the doctor, you expect to describe your symptoms, be examined and possibly be sent for some tests to find out what is happening to you. This may or may not happen at the initial visit. It could be spread over a number of visits. The biggest clues that aid a doctor in trying to answer the questions above are found in the story or *history* of the illness. This includes both the symptoms that have developed and, less obviously, the symptoms that are not there. It also, very importantly, includes the time line of how these symptoms developed. The importance placed on each symptom may be different for the patient and the doctor. See the example on the next page.

Example: Anne's story

Anne has had increasing symptoms for some time but has been unable to go to work for the last two weeks because of severe tiredness. She goes to see her family doctor (Dr Andrews).

Anne spends a long time with her doctor and tells her all about how she's been feeling. Anne gets the feeling that the doctor is not very interested in her tiredness and is annoyed because that's her worst symptom. She feels that Dr Andrews is asking a lot of questions about symptoms that are less troublesome and even asking about things she doesn't have. Anne leaves the surgery with a sick note and an appointment for two weeks' time.

Example: Dr Andrews' story

Dr Andrews is in her morning clinic. Her first patient is Anne. Anne describes her tiredness in great detail.

Dr Andrews knows that tiredness is a very common symptom in a large number of illnesses and so this does not really help her to make a decision about what is wrong with Anne. She asks questions that will give her more useful information as she has some ideas of what might be wrong.

Dr Andrews has ruled out a number of illnesses by Anne's answers and signs her off work for a further two weeks. However, Anne seems frustrated when she leaves.

Diagnosis is a process of reducing a large number of possibilities to a shorter list. The most useful information may lie in those symptoms that are rare or very specific to a particular illness rather than those which are common to lots of illnesses. Indeed some symptoms occur in healthy people. These may not be obvious, but are significant to the doctor.

Certain symptoms occur in groups which may point the doctor to a certain diagnosis. If one symptom is missing it may rule out that particular diagnosis.

People can read articles about illnesses in magazines, books or on the internet. These often give lists of symptoms that look very similar to how a person feels and may lead them to think that they have that illness. However, such lists do not show which symptoms are more important or the time line in which they will develop. As a result they can be very misleading.

What happens next?

At this stage, the doctor will have a few possibilities in mind, which can be reduced further by examination and the results of tests. People often find it surprising that tests are less important than they imagine. Usually a doctor will have a good idea of a likely diagnosis. Tests may be ordered to exclude rare but serious illnesses that seem unlikely but important not to miss. Such tests are expected to be normal. Also, some tests may be helpful in certain situations but not in others.

> KEY POINT
>
> **Are tests helpful? If epilepsy is a possibility a test called an EEG (electroencephalography) may be done. If the EEG is abnormal epilepsy is likely. Often, however, it is normal so this does not help the doctor make a diagnosis one way or the other. People can have a normal EEG and still have epilepsy. Doctors have learnt it is the history that makes the diagnosis rather than the tests. This is true of many other neurological conditions.**

Sometimes there are two different tests that will give the same information, so only one will need to be done. This is why you might wonder why you had one test while someone else you know had another for what seemed the same symptoms.

Many people with neurological symptoms will expect to go for a 'scan'. As described above, these will rarely show anything abnormal that is not already suspected by the neurologist. Sometimes people feel that having a scan would help them feel more certain. It can be difficult to believe the doctors when they say a scan isn't necessary. But they are trying to prevent unnecessary stress for you, for example while waiting for the test and results. The same is true of having repeat scans 'just to be sure'.

The other questions

All this leads to a diagnosis and answers the question 'What is it?' In turn, this can help to answer other questions of treatment and prognosis. A harder question sometimes is 'What caused it?' In some illnesses the cause is known. In others there may be ongoing research and in others still, even less is known. However, an illness may be diagnosed and treatment advised even when its cause is not fully understood. Multiple sclerosis or MS is a good example of such a situation. Doctors can be sure of the diagnosis even though they still don't know fully what causes it.

> KEY POINT
>
> **The lack of explanation for symptoms can be very frustrating. However, it is important not to let it prevent you from working on a treatment.**

SECTION 3: How the brain and body work

This section will explain how some parts of the body work. Some of the information may be familiar to you and other parts may be new. Many people with symptoms find it useful to understand more about how their body works and how the various systems link together.

The nervous system

What is it and what does it do?

The nervous system is made up of the brain, the spinal cord and the peripheral nerves. The brain and the spinal cord are together known as the central nervous system (CNS). Nerves radiate out from the CNS to every part of the body. These nerves are known as the peripheral nervous system (Figure 2.1).

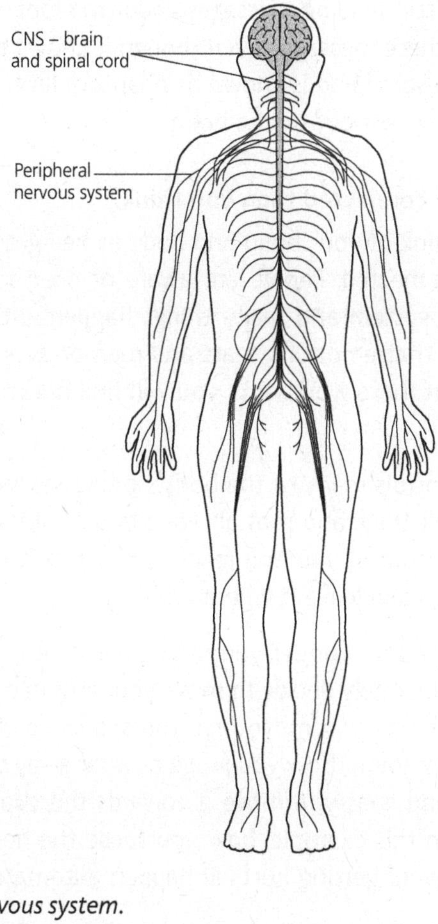

Figure 2.1 Parts of the nervous system.

The nervous system moves messages around the body. These messages run through the nerves in a similar way to electricity through power lines. They are very fast: more than 250 miles per hour! Special chemicals or 'neurotransmitters' pass messages from one nerve to another.

The brain sends messages out to the body to tell it what to do – move, swallow, change heart rate, etc. The nerves also bring information back to the brain from the rest of the body. This tells the brain what the body is doing and also what is happening around us. This information is gathered by specially adapted nerve cells. As well as the well-known 'senses', there are others that may not be so familiar – temperature, pain, vibration and the sense of where your body parts (such as hands or legs) are. The brain links all this information together and makes decisions about what to tell the body to do next.

In some situations this system may become confused. This can be due to disease or injury interrupting the nerves or damaging part of the brain. It may also be caused by the wrong messages being sent through an otherwise healthy system. Let's look at an example of this: people who have had part of their leg amputated. For many years after the amputation, many people complain of pain and other sensations in the foot that is missing. The nerves are still sending messages about the foot which is no longer there. The brain still believes these messages even though it knows the foot is missing. Such pain can be very troublesome and is known as phantom limb pain. This is an example of wrong messages being sent out by the brain.

Brain and body – more connected than you think?

Sometimes you may think of your brain and body as being quite separate things but they are very much connected. People are aware of only a tiny amount of all the activity in the nervous system and many things happen automatically. What is not so obvious, however, is that emotions, fears and memories are also found within the nervous system. Later in these workbooks you will find out more about how all these link together.

The nervous system controls many of the body's processes. We are aware of some of these but most we don't think about at all. For example, imagine you are thirsty and there is a cup of tea in front of you. You reach out to pick it up but the handle is hot and so you quickly let go and leave it where it is.

At first glance this might seem under your conscious control. You are aware you can see the cup and you deliberately decide to move your arm to pick it up. What you don't think about is which muscle you move first, the sequence in which you move your shoulder, elbow and wrist joints, how you judge how far away the cup is, how you keep track of where your hand is as you move it towards the cup and, most importantly of all, for your safety. In this example, how you sense the heat and in a split second remove your hand to avoid getting hurt, all happen automatically but are still under the control of your nervous system. The quick removal of the hand is known as a **reflex action**.

Another example is how the nervous system controls breathing. Breathing usually happens without people thinking about it but one can override this. This will be discussed further in the section on the respiratory/breathing system.

Autonomic nervous system

The *autonomic nervous system* controls the heart rate, breathing, blood pressure and the way the digestive system works. There are two parts to it which have opposite actions: the *sympathetic nervous system*, which reacts to stress, and the *parasympathetic nervous system*, which relaxes us. Our stress system is balanced by our relaxation system. They have opposite effects on the body.

Imagine that the body is like a car – then the sympathetic system would be the accelerator and the parasympathetic system would be the brakes. You can't press on both at the same time. In the same way both of these parts of the nervous system can't be active at the same time.

If you press on the accelerator, the car speeds up. To slow it down there are two choices, take your foot off the accelerator or press on the brakes, or often both of these at once. Or in body terms: stop the stress reaction or increase the relaxation system.

Usually the body can cope quickly with changes in the balance between the stress system and the relaxation system, and rapidly return things back to normal. As these systems balance the heart rate, breathing, bowels and bladder, this explains how these systems are commonly affected at times of stress.

The fight or flight adrenaline response

This is the body's response to danger, fear or threat. It is a normal response to frightening or dangerous things such as being woken from sleep by a noise in the middle of the night. The body reacts to a combination of messages from the nervous system (as described above) and a chemical called adrenaline in the blood. At the time this happens you may not really be aware of it going on but afterwards you might notice that your heart is beating faster or your hands are shaking.

What does the fight or flight adrenaline response do?

It basically prepares a person to either stand up and fight or to run away (Figure 2.2). The heart rate gets faster to increase blood flow round the body. Blood goes to places where it is needed most, for example away from the skin, hands, feet and stomach, and into the muscles. The saliva dries up and the gut slows down. The muscles tense to prepare to act, and the skin starts to sweat to cool the body for running. Breathing becomes faster and deeper to provide the person with more oxygen. The pupils dilate/

widen to look for danger and the person becomes more alert. Finally, our body reacts to provide us with more energy from its sugar reserves.

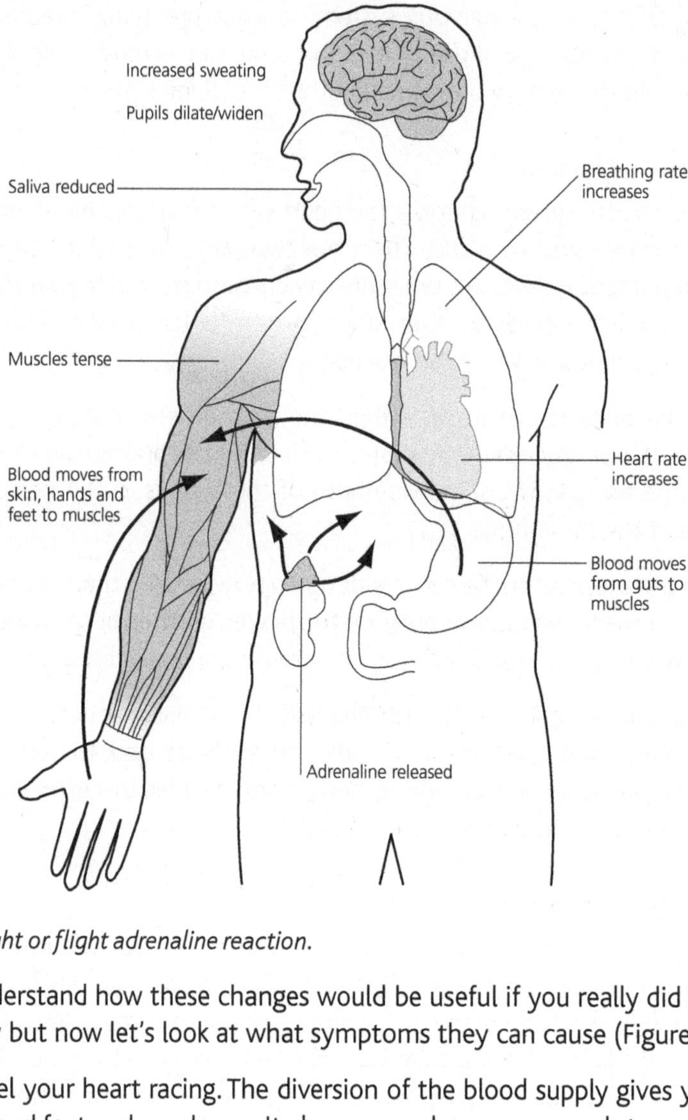

Figure 2.2 Fight or flight adrenaline reaction.

We can understand how these changes would be useful if you really did have to fight or run away but now let's look at what symptoms they can cause (Figure 2.3).

You may feel your heart racing. The diversion of the blood supply gives you cold skin, cold hands and feet and numbness. It also can produce nausea and stomach heaviness. Your tummy may churn. The changes in your breathing may cause you to feel short of breath, with sensations of choking, dizziness and chest pains. You can also get symptoms of hyperventilation/over-breathing (see later). You find yourself sweating and with a dry mouth due to lack of saliva. The changes in your eyes may be strong enough to blur your vision. Feeling alert to danger can make a person feel on edge. It can also make you react to the slightest noise or minor irritation. The tension in your muscles causes aches and pains. You can also experience an urge to run and feel tired and drained afterwards.

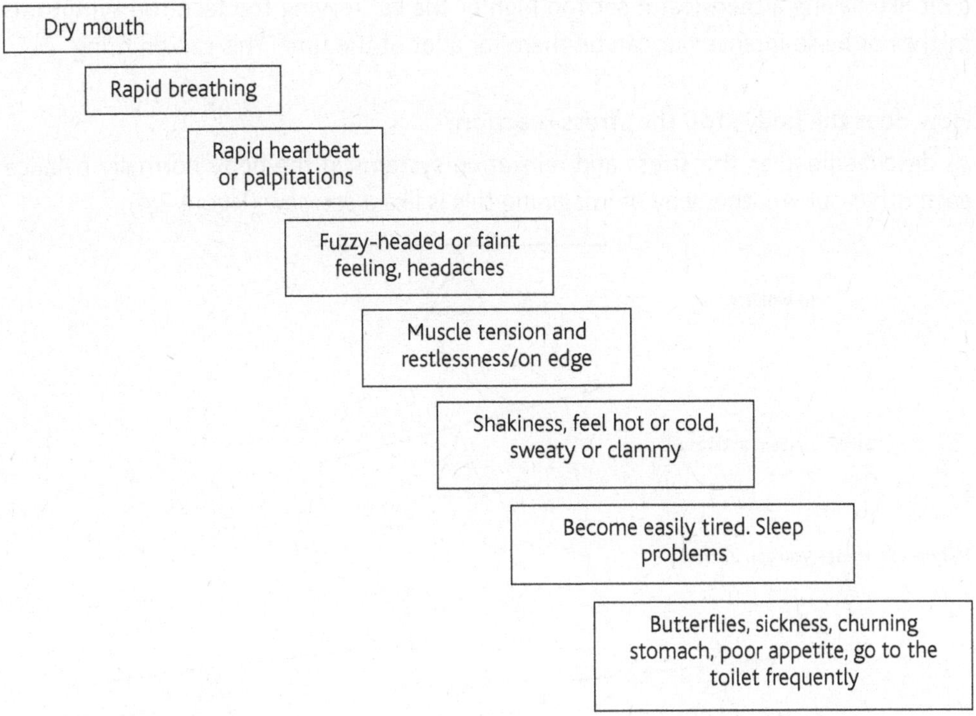

Figure 2.3 Common physical reactions in the fight or flight adrenaline response.

Panic attacks and anxiety

Panic attacks are an extremely sudden and very intense version of this 'fight or flight' adrenaline reaction. It is as if the stress system has been set off by mistake. The symptoms that result can be frightening to experience. Your heart races, you can't breathe, you may have pain across your chest and you feel an overwhelming urge to escape. There is a fear that something dreadful is going to happen and some people even think they might die.

Panic attacks are very common. Each year almost one in 10 people will experience a panic attack. You might even have experienced one yourself at some time. Luckily, these panic attacks are usually short-lived as the body runs low on adrenaline quite quickly. However, sometimes panic attacks can reoccur. As these attacks are so scary, it is quite common to become scared of having the panic attacks themselves. People can start to avoid any situations or events where they fear the panic may occur and so the situation gets even worse.

Sometimes the stress reaction happens when there is nothing obvious to fear. It may be triggered by something you are thinking or even seem to be out of the blue. In other people it may seem as if the system is constantly firing off for very little cause. It is a bit like having a thermostat set too high or the car revving too fast. The symptoms might not be so intense but can be there for a lot of the time. This can be tiring.

How does the body stop the stress reaction?

As described earlier, the stress and relaxation systems in the body normally balance each other out. Another way of imagining this is like a see-saw (Figure 2.4).

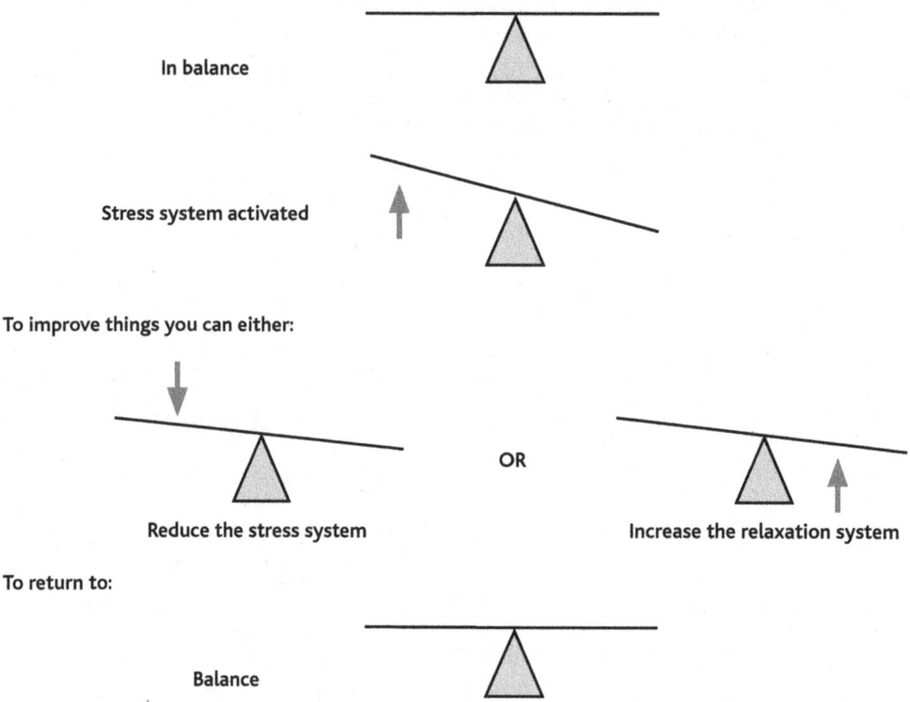

Figure 2.4 The balancing act between stress and relaxation.

To learn ways to boost your relaxation system, see the Toolbox.

> **KEY POINT**
> **The 'fight or flight' symptoms can make you feel uncomfortable or unwell. However, they are not dangerous.**

Sometimes, chronic (lasting a long time) stress may cause these symptoms to be there for a lot of the time. The more a person notices their body's reaction, the more they worry about it and this can make it worse. Unfortunately, people may not notice what set this reaction off, and only notice how they feel physically. If you can recognise this, it can help you to change it.

It might be difficult to imagine how your thoughts can affect what you feel. Let's think for a minute about how someone on a roller coaster might feel: perhaps heart pounding, breathless, stomach flipping, gripping the safety bar and maybe even shouting out loud? So is that excitement or is it fear? Or is it a bit of both? People are all different in how they respond to such situations. Two different people may finish the ride with quite different feelings – one white with fear vowing never to go back on it, and the other running to join the queue again. What it certainly involves is adrenaline and the stress system. Your heart may beat faster in both fearful and exciting situations but how you feel about it may be completely different. Workbook 3 will cover more about the interaction between how you feel physically and how you think.

The respiratory system

What is it and what does it do?

The respiratory/breathing system (Figure 2.5) itself is made up of the nose, mouth, trachea (windpipe) and the lungs. You breathe in oxygen from the air and it is taken to where it is needed in the body. You breathe out carbon dioxide, which the body produces when it burns energy.

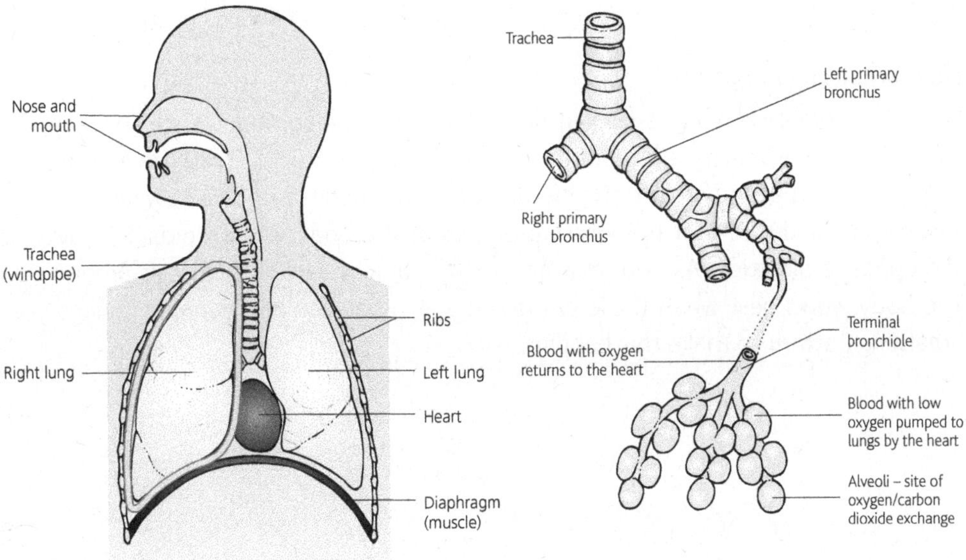

Figure 2.5 The respiratory system.

The lungs are surrounded by the chest cavity. This can be thought of as a kind of flexible box made up of the bones and muscles of the ribcage (Figure 2.6). The base of this box is a large muscle called the diaphragm and the top involves the muscles and bones of the neck and shoulders.

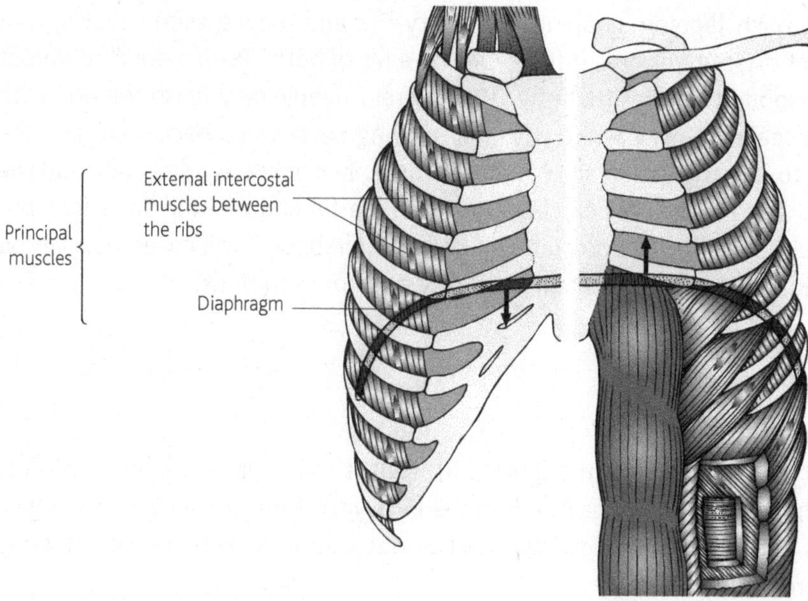

Figure 2.6 The rib cage.

How breathing happens

When you breathe in, air is sucked down the windpipe to your lungs. This happens because the chest cavity around the lungs expands (Figure 2.7). Once the air is in your lungs, oxygen is absorbed into the bloodstream and then transported away to be used all over the body. One of the waste products of the body, carbon dioxide, travels in the opposite direction. As you breathe out, it is blown back into the air around you. The body works best when these two gases are in balance and you can change your breathing pattern to make this happen.

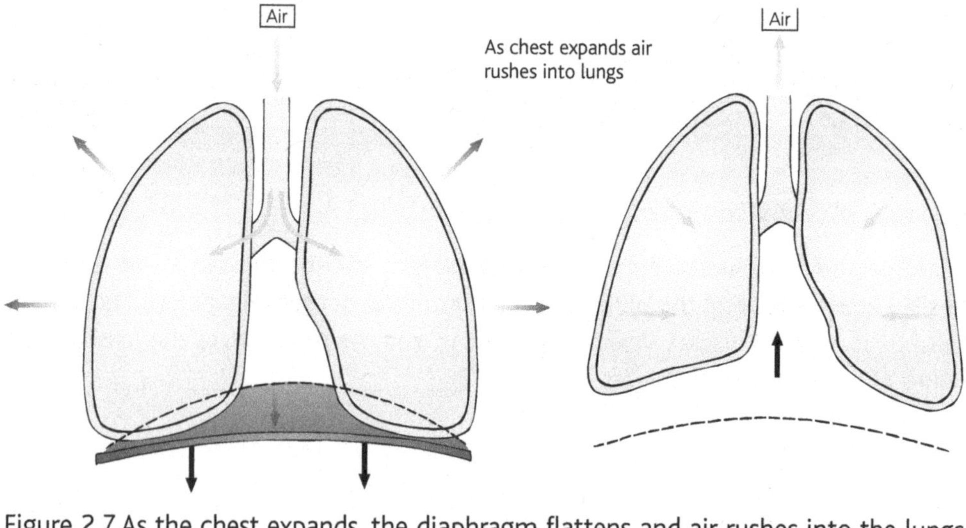

Figure 2.7 As the chest expands, the diaphragm flattens and air rushes into the lungs.

The diaphragm is the main muscle that helps your lungs to work when you are resting and breathing normally. As it tenses and moves downwards it makes the chest cavity bigger and the lungs expand and suck in air. When it relaxes, the chest cavity gets smaller and it squeezes the unwanted carbon dioxide out. This is known as **abdominal, relaxed breathing**.

Another way of increasing the space in the chest is by using the neck and chest muscles to raise the shoulders. This takes more effort. It can be useful at times when you need to breathe harder. A good example of this is when you exercise. This is called **thoracic breathing**.

Mostly you breathe without thinking about it. Sometimes you get out of breath and then you may notice your breathing more. You can also control your breathing on purpose at times, for example when holding the breath underwater or blowing out the candles on a birthday cake. People are able to change both the speed and the depth of their breathing for a short time. But doing this for longer would begin to become uncomfortable as the body starts to notice the changes in the oxygen and carbon dioxide levels.

If you start to breathe faster, you tend to take short, shallow breaths which blow away more carbon dioxide. This is called **hyperventilation**. Sometimes you may do this without noticing and, over a period of time, it can cause uncomfortable symptoms. This type of breathing tends to occur when we feel anxious and stressed. This is covered in more detail later in this workbook.

The motor/movement system

This consists of the bones, the joints between them and the ligaments and muscles that surround them (see figure below). It also involves the nerves that tell the muscles when to move and that feed information back to the nervous system about what is happening to the body.

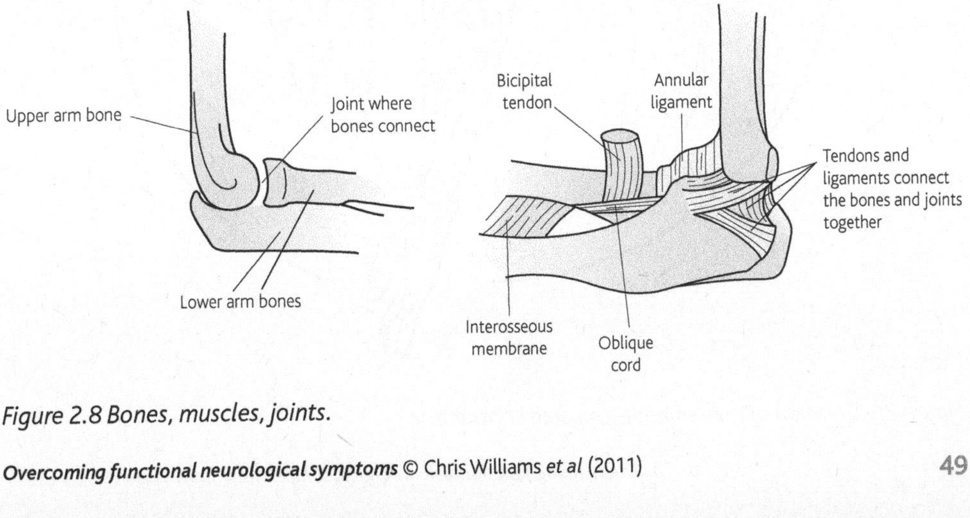

Figure 2.8 Bones, muscles, joints.

The muscles are important to the joints, both for movement and for support. Movements may be under a person's conscious or unconscious control. Let's consider again the previous example about reaching out to pick up a cup of tea. Although you consciously decide to carry out the action, you certainly don't think about each muscle separately or about which joint (finger, wrist, elbow or shoulder) to move first. Such combinations of movements are learned by the body and become second nature with practice, although may seem very difficult at first as any baby would tell you!

How the body moves

To bend a joint, the muscles around it need to become shorter or *contract*. The opposite happens when the muscles *relax* or get longer (Figure 2.9). Most joints will have two sets of muscles around them which can pull in opposite directions to move back and forth.

The two sets may not be equal in strength and some movements will be easier than others.

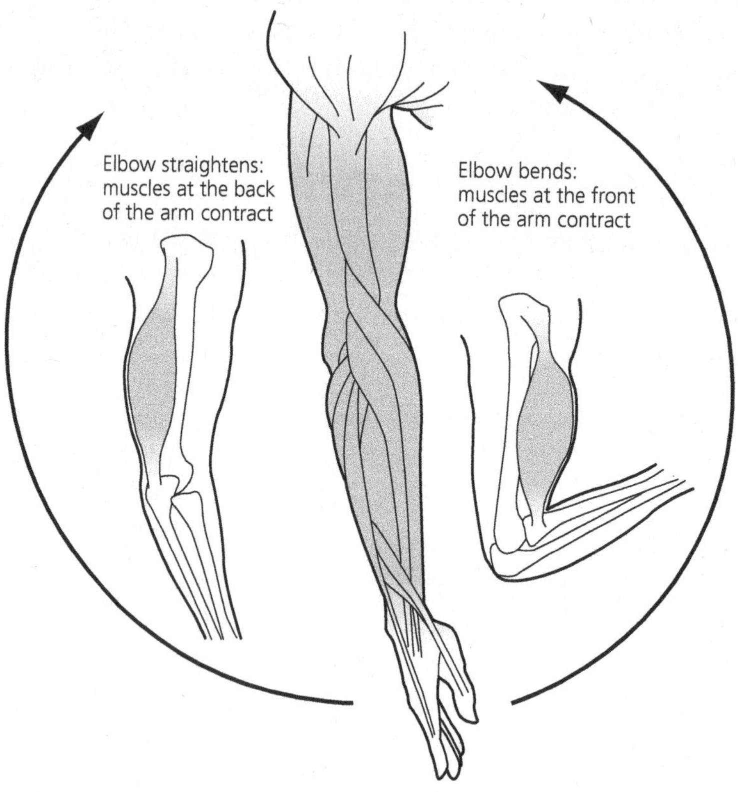

Figure 2.9 Creation of movement by muscle contraction.

There is always some tension in the muscles to keep the joint in a certain position. Sometimes this may be uneven. This might cause the joint to be held differently than usual. If this is prolonged the muscles can begin to ache. If any parts of a joint are injured or irritated then the muscles nearby may shorten automatically and go into *spasm* (Figure 2.10). This may be very painful.

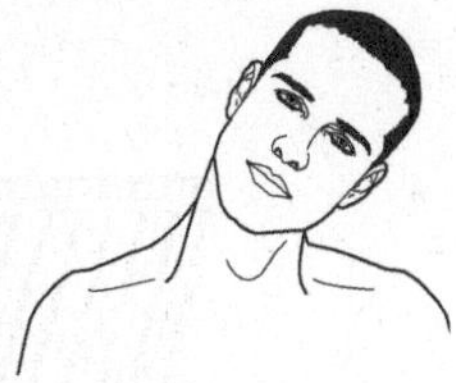

Figure 2.10 Illustration of a neck muscle spasm.

If you have ever had a stiff neck, you might remember how difficult and painful it was to try to straighten it up. This happens to protect the injured part and allow it time to heal.

Muscles are made up of lots of tiny muscle fibres which slide across each other to shorten or lengthen the muscle (Figure 2.11).

Muscles can be built up with use, both from deliberate exercise or everyday movements. For example, most right-handed people will have bigger arm muscles on the right than the left just from using that arm more often. Muscles can also get weak from lack of use. This can happen very quickly. For example, someone who had a broken leg in a plaster cast would notice that their leg muscles had become much thinner and weaker when the cast is taken off just six weeks later.

Over time muscles 'learn' positions that feel comfortable to the person. Try this experiment.

Experiment

Cross your arms in front of your chest as you would normally do in everyday life. Now try to cross them the opposite way. Put the arm that is usually on top under the other one, or move the one that is usually on the outside to the inside. Is it easy? Does it feel the same? Do you have to think more about doing it?

Most people will find one way fairly natural and comfortable but find the other feels 'odd' or more difficult to do. This happens throughout the body. Mostly this makes no difference to a person. Sometimes, however, you can 'learn' positions of muscles or joints that can actually cause you discomfort in the long run. This will be covered in more detail later in the workbook.

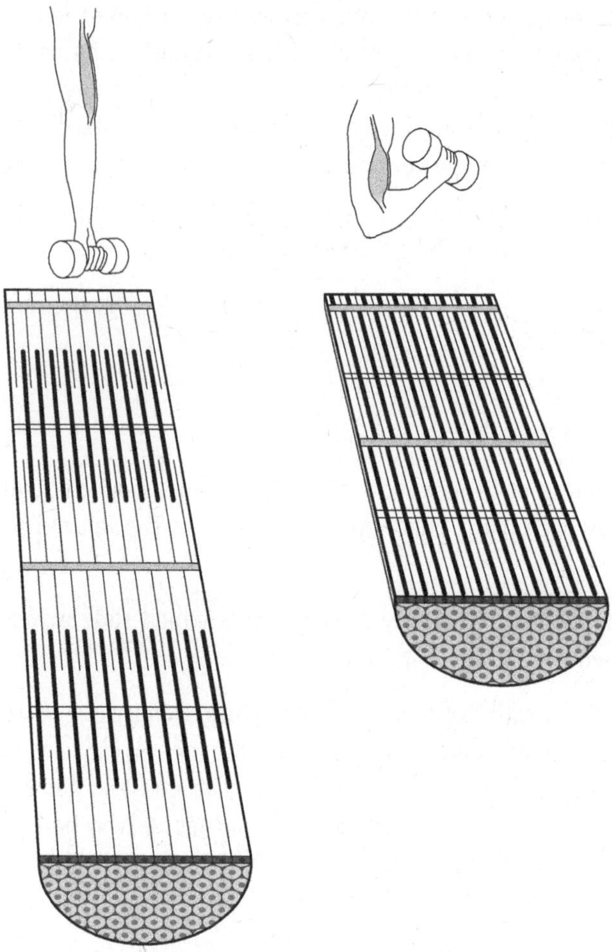

Figure 2.11 The muscle fibres: relaxed (left) and contracted (right).

Muscles can stop working properly for a number of reasons – due to disease, injury or even their patterns of use. This will in turn affect how you use your joints and how you can move around.

How people use their muscles

Sometimes the way people tend to use muscles can cause pain or discomfort. This can be direct or indirect. It is obvious that repeated use of a muscle may cause pain afterwards. Going on a long hill walk might make your muscles ache the next day or so, especially if a person isn't used to it. Another cause of discomfort is increased tension within the muscles. Writer's cramp causes pain because of the prolonged grip on the pen as well as the movements in the hand and wrist. It is another more subtle form of overuse. A less obvious cause of increased muscle tension is stress. For example, if someone is anxious, they tend to tense up the muscles even when they are 'at rest'. This can directly cause aches and pains all over the body without any increased exercise or activity at all.

Sometimes people talk about 'posture' or how you hold your body. If people mention 'good posture', you tend to think of standing up straight and tall. When they talk of 'bad posture', you may imagine people slouched over or slumped. You may feel that somehow 'good posture' is better for you in some way but in reality people often feel more comfortable slumped.

Imagine someone sitting at a computer keyboard. For a short time it doesn't really matter how they type. Most people will sit in the way they feel most comfortable, 'good' or otherwise. However, if they are working for longer, they might start to ache and feel stiff in the neck and shoulders and over time they may develop more chronic pain. Eventually they will look for ways to avoid these pains – perhaps changing their desk height or their chair, buying special rests for their wrists or other such devices. The bad posture feels better in the short term but, in the long run, good posture can be protective.

Often though, it is not so obvious that 'posture' is affecting a person in this way. As mentioned above, following an injury to a joint, the muscles around it may go into spasm to protect it and allow time for healing. This is a reflex which you can't control. However, you can also try to protect the injured part in a more conscious way. You may try to hold the joint still. This is called 'learned guarding' and avoids the possibility of further pain or injury. If it continues it may cause disuse of the affected side (a little like the example of the broken leg) and over-activity of the opposite side.

Over time this disuse can affect the muscles so that when you do try to use them again they are weak and do not work properly. This is called 'learned weakness'. The over-activity of the opposite side may then cause discomfort in the unaffected muscles. This is quite common in people with back pain but may be difficult to spot. Unfortunately, if someone develop these habits it will usually take longer to get better. It can become a vicious circle. The more the person tries to avoid pain, the more pain they get. It can also begin to affect other parts of their body and sometimes can go on so long that the person may almost forget the original injury that started the whole process off.

As you have seen, anxiety can increase tension in your muscles. It is easy to see how this might add to this process. In addition, a person is more likely to guard a painful area if they believe that they might make the situation worse. In this way anxiety or worrying can actually increase pain.

Thus your emotions, posture and movements may all interact to affect how your motor system works. Since your nervous system also has an important part to play in controlling your motor system, any factors that affect one may also affect the other. This may help to explain how some functional neurological symptoms develop or are made worse as the body adapts to them.

Hyperventilation

Hyperventilation is a change in the breathing pattern which can cause symptoms throughout your body. It is very common and may affect almost one in 10 people on a regular basis. Nearly everyone has experienced short episodes of hyperventilation during stressful events and could recognise some of the description below.

Example: Jane has hyperventilation

Jane is scared of large dogs. She is walking across the park one day when one runs straight towards her, barking. She stands frozen to the spot and begins to breathe faster. She is breathing short, shallow breaths through her mouth and notices her chest moving in and out. Her heart is beating faster. Jane feels breathless and panicked. She begins to feel a bit dizzy and her mouth seems dry. Her vision begins to blur and she notices a tight feeling across her chest. Her fingers and hands begin to tingle and she feels more and more dizzy. She barely notices the dog's owner rushing over. He calls the dog back to him. The dog stops barking and runs to him immediately. He apologises profusely to Jane. She is quite shaken but able to talk and reassures him that she is okay. Her breathing slows down and returns to normal. Within a couple of minutes her symptoms wear off completely.

The symptoms of **long-term** hyperventilation are much harder to spot but can have a major effect on some people.

In Section 1 of this workbook you filled in a list of all your symptoms. We are now going to take a closer look at these to see if hyperventilation could be playing a part in your own symptoms.

Please use the checklist below.

Symptom checklist

Symptom	*Do you notice many of these symptoms?*	
Chest pain	Yes ☐	No ☐
Feeling tense	Yes ☐	No ☐
Blurred vision	Yes ☐	No ☐
Dizziness	Yes ☐	No ☐
Confusion or loss of touch with reality	Yes ☐	No ☐
Fast or deep breathing	Yes ☐	No ☐
Shortness of breath	Yes ☐	No ☐
Tightness across chest	Yes ☐	No ☐

Symptom	*Do you notice many of these symptoms?*	
Bloated sensation in stomach	Yes ☐	No ☐
Tingling in fingers and hands	Yes ☐	No ☐
Difficulty breathing/taking a deep breath	Yes ☐	No ☐
Stiffness or cramps in fingers and hands	Yes ☐	No ☐
Tightness around the mouth	Yes ☐	No ☐
Cold hands or feet	Yes ☐	No ☐
Palpitations in the chest	Yes ☐	No ☐
Anxiety	Yes ☐	No ☐

If you have ticked many of the symptoms in this checklist and notice these at times you feel panicky you might like to read more about hyperventilation and how it can affect your body. You may also benefit from trying some of the breathing exercises in Toolbox D.

If you are unsure whether hyperventilation is affecting you, you might like to try the following experiment.

Optional experiment

This is a forced exercise in overbreathing. It might make you feel uncomfortable but it should not be dangerous. Sometimes the symptoms can make you scared. If you are at all worried about this, try to do it when there is someone else around. If you have asthma or other chronic breathing problems you may want to ask your doctor before you try this. Also please don't do this if you are pregnant or have epilepsy.

Sit and breathe deeply through your mouth as if you are running. Try to do this for at least 30 seconds. Most people will start to develop unpleasant symptoms within this time. If your own troublesome symptoms seem to flare up during this, it is likely that hyperventilation has a part to play in your own situation.

More about hyperventilation

Hyperventilation syndrome has two different forms, sudden or acute onset and a more everyday, chronic form. The sudden form comes on rapidly and has more intense symptoms. It is often associated with anxiety and panic. Sometimes people are not aware of what triggers it and just experience the unpleasant and rather frightening symptoms it causes. The more long-term, chronic form causes similar but milder symptoms. It is really a 'bad habit' of breathing. Most people with this type of hyperventilation will notice the symptoms it causes, but are often unaware of the underlying change in their breathing pattern.

How does it cause these symptoms?

These symptoms are mainly caused by changes in the carbon dioxide levels in the blood (see Figure 2.12). As described in the section on the respiratory system above, these short, shallow breaths cause you to breathe out more carbon dioxide than usual and so the amount left in your blood stream is reduced. This has effects on the brain causing **confusion**, **agitation** and **anxiety**, **dizziness** or even **fainting** and **depersonalisation symptoms** (see p. 58). It can cause **heart palpitation** too.

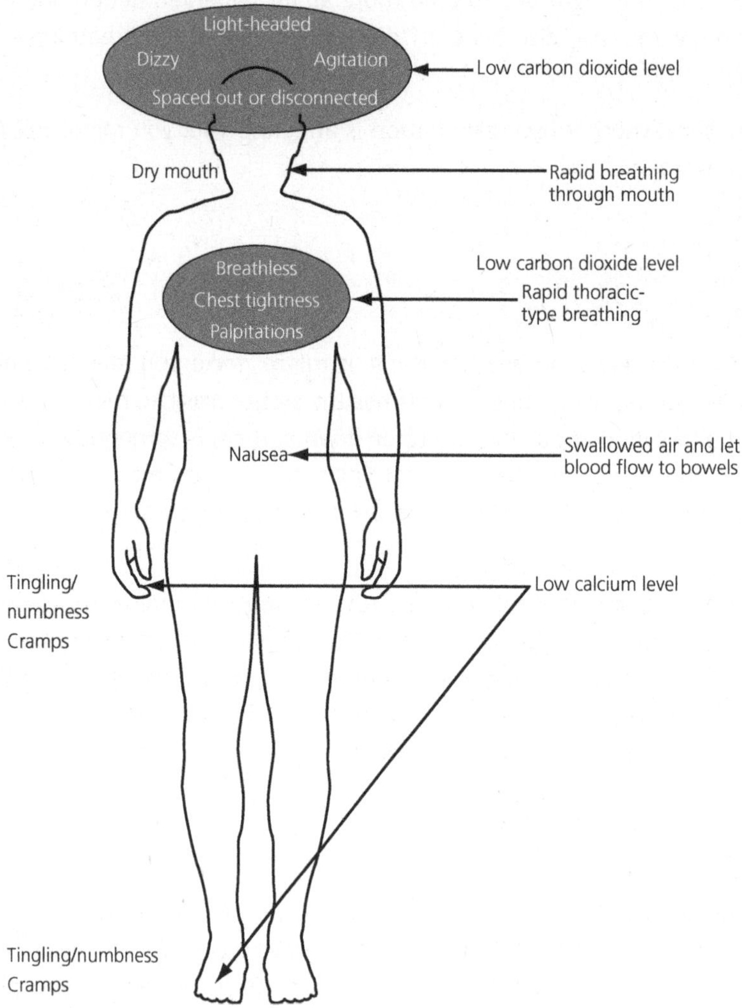

Figure 2.12 Acute hyperventilation.

It also has an effect on the levels of calcium in the blood. When the calcium level in the blood falls, it affects the working of the nervous system. This leads to **numbness and tingling** (especially in the hands and feet, and around the mouth and nose). It can also cause **muscles to twitch** and even **spasms** or **cramps in your hands and feet**.

The lowered carbon dioxide levels may cause the lungs to **wheeze**. The extra effort of breathing makes the person feel **short of breath** and, because of the tendency to switch to thoracic breathing, people can get **pains or tenderness in the chest**. You are more likely to breathe through your mouth during hyperventilation as it is very difficult to breathe fast through your nose for very long. This mouth breathing can cause a **dry mouth**.

The more chronic type of overbreathing causes similar symptoms. In addition, some people **yawn and sigh** more than other people seem to. Or they might have an **irritable cough** or clear their throats more than usual. Sometimes you get a feeling that you **need to take a deep breath**. It can cause **tiredness**, **lack of concentration** and **sleep disturbances** too. Sometimes there are particularly **vivid dreams or nightmares**. There may be **episodes of weakness and exhaustion** during the day. These seem to happen for no obvious reason. The constant use of thoracic breathing may cause **muscular aches** and **tension around the neck, shoulders and jaw**. When people hyperventilate they might also swallow excessive air. This can cause **bloating, burping, nausea** and uncomfortable **pressure feelings in our stomachs**.

What can be done about this?

The first step is to consider whether hyperventilation may be affecting you and causing some of your symptoms. It is unlikely to be the only thing that is happening to you but it can certainly worsen your existing situation. This is particularly the case with the everyday, chronic type of overbreathing as you are unlikely to be aware of it. Luckily, it is a pattern of breathing that develops as a 'bad habit' rather than because of an underlying illness. There are ways to 'un-learn' this pattern of breathing. There are various methods to train people to breathe in a more relaxed way again. You can find out more about these in Toolbox D.

Depersonalisation: feeling cut-off and disconnected from things

Depersonalisation is a strange experience felt by many people at one time or another. It is a feeling of unreality and disconnection from your usual self. This can last from a matter of seconds to hours, days or even weeks. It may come and go without warning. Depersonalisation is a symptom of a variety of different conditions and can also happen to healthy people too. It is often accompanied by another symptom called **derealisation**. This is when the world around you also appears unfamiliar.

It can be quite difficult to describe what this feels like and often people don't talk about it very much. Many have said 'I just don't feel like me' or that they feel numb. It may feel like walking around with a goldfish bowl on your head, or as if your head is full of cotton wool. It can feel very disturbing. Someone described it as 'losing your sense of being alive'. Some worry what others will think about them or even that they are 'going mad'.

What does it feel like?

There are many 'funny' experiences that might be part of depersonalisation/derealisation. Below is a checklist of some of the most common descriptions that people have given. Some of them may seem quite bizarre to you. As many as possible have been included as there is a huge range of different experiences so, even if you have only one or two, you may still have depersonalisation/derealisation.

Out of the blue, I feel strange, as if I were not real or as if I were cut off from the world	☐
What I see looks 'flat' or 'lifeless' as if I were looking at a picture	☐
Parts of my body feel as if they don't belong to me	☐
While doing something I have the feeling of being a 'detached observer' of myself	☐
My body feels very light, as if it were floating on air	☐
I have the feeling of not having any thoughts at all, so that when I speak it feels as if my words were uttered by an 'automaton'	☐
Familiar voices (including my own) sound remote and unreal	☐
I have the feeling that my hands or my feet have become larger or smaller	☐
My surroundings feel detached or unreal, as if there was a veil between me and the outside world	☐
It seems as if things I have recently done had taken place a long time ago. For example, anything which I have done this morning feels as if it were done weeks ago	☐
I feel detached from memories of things that have happened to me, as if I had not been involved in them	☐
Objects around me seem to look smaller or further away	☐
I cannot feel properly the objects that I touch with my hands; it feels as if it were not me who was touching it	☐
I do not seem able to picture things in my mind, for example the face of a close friend or a familiar place	☐
When a part of my body hurts, I feel so detached from the pain that it feels as if it were 'somebody else's pain'	☐
I have the feeling of being outside my body	☐

When I move it doesn't feel as if I were in charge of the movements, so that I feel 'automatic' and mechanical as if I were a 'robot'	☐
The smell of things no longer gives me a feeling of pleasure or dislike	☐
I feel so detached from my thoughts that they seem to have a 'life' of their own	☐
I have to touch myself to make sure that I have a body or a real existence	☐
I seem to have lost some bodily sensations (e.g. of hunger or thirst) so that when I eat or drink, it feels an automatic routine	☐

Some of these descriptions may seem familiar to you and some might sound quite unfamiliar. Some may occur also in other conditions as well as being symptoms of depersonalisation. Everyone has a slightly different experience of depersonalisation/derealisation but often there will be some similarities.

What can cause depersonalisation/derealisation?

It might be surprising to discover that these types of symptoms are actually quite common. Studies have shown that up to one in two people will have them at some point in their lives. Some situations can make these symptoms more likely. These include being very tired, being very frightened or feeling very stressed. Some people find that having caffeine or alcohol might worsen their symptoms.

Infections such as colds and flu may cause temporary depersonalisation symptoms. Many people feel 'spacey' and 'not quite there' when they've been laid up in bed with such illnesses. These symptoms can also happen in a number of other illnesses including epilepsy, migraines and when blood sugar falls too low in diabetes.

Depersonalisation symptoms are also common in a number of disorders such as depression and anxiety. They are especially frequent where there is marked anxiety or panic. They may also happen as side effects of certain medicines, including some anti-depressants. Some people notice that they can be brought on by upsetting thoughts or flashbacks, especially if there has been a distressing event or trauma in the past.

Hyperventilation (see previous section) is a common cause of depersonalisation symptoms. These can be very unpleasant and quite frightening when combined with all the other physical symptoms that hyperventilation can cause.

What can be done about it?

Knowing more about these symptoms and how common they are can be very reassuring. It may make it easier to explain to the people around us so that they can understand how strange one can feel at times.

Often people can identify the cause, such as medicine side effects or lack of sleep, which can be tackled to improve these symptoms. But sometimes people may not be able to exactly pinpoint what is causing them. But often the symptoms will reduce as you begin to recover from your other symptoms. Using the CBT (cognitive behavioural therapy or talking therapy) approach can help too.

Sometimes, if the symptoms are very prolonged or frequent, more specialist help may be needed. If this is the case then you might like to discuss it further with your own doctor or nurse.

SECTION 4: Difficulties with uncertainty

As mentioned earlier in this workbook, when people become ill, they face a number of uncertainties and questions. Seeking advice from your doctor might answer some of these but often you might be left with yet more questions. Let's look at John's story.

Example: John's problem

John is helping his daughter move house. He injures his elbow picking up a heavy box but it seems only minor at the time and he carries on for the rest of the afternoon. The next morning it is very sore and he cannot do up the buttons on his shirt. He takes the day off work and the following day, with little improvement, he goes to see his doctor. The doctor tells him that there does not appear to be a serious injury and advises him to rest it and take some ibuprofen. He thinks it will settle down over the next few days. John asks about a sling but the doctor does not think this is necessary.

John takes the rest of the week off work. He buys an elasticated bandage as he had used one on his knee in the past. This seems to help. He tries hard not to move his arm and finds it helps to keep it held still across his chest. He eats his food one-handed and his wife helps him get dressed. Whenever he takes the bandage off his elbow seems to hurt and feels very strange. He also notices his shoulder beginning to ache. John is convinced he has done more damage than the doctor first suspected. He is worried that he might make it worse. After two weeks he makes another appointment to see his doctor.

The doctor examines him again and tries to reassure John. He suggests that John should try to use his arm normally. John knows his elbow is sore and stiff and that moving it seems to make this worse. He asks for an X-ray but the doctor disagrees. He does, however, give John a sick note as his job involves carrying parcels and files.

Over the next few weeks John feels his arm is becoming thinner. Although the sharp pain is less, it aches and is very stiff. He notices that he cannot straighten his arm any more. He avoids using it as much as possible. His work colleague phones him to ask when he will return. He can't see how he can do his job and so stays signed off. He feels very miserable. He worries that he will never get better and will have to give up his job.

Eventually he returns to the doctor. This time the doctor finds that examination is not normal. John's muscles are wasted, his arm is weak and his elbow cannot move normally. The doctor explains that he thinks this is not due to the original injury but to the lack of use that happened afterwards. John finds this difficult to believe but he is keen to try anything that might help. The doctor suggests a referral to a physiotherapist. John has a friend who had physiotherapy for a football injury which was very successful and so agrees to try this.

The physiotherapist shows John how to do exercises with his arm. She reassures him that he cannot make things worse and explains how muscles and joints work. John feels more reassured. He tries the exercises and feels things improving. After a couple of months of exercises his arm returns to normal. He is able to return to work and has no further problems with his elbow.

What could have helped?

What happened to John was very unfortunate but not uncommon. There was an interaction between John's beliefs (that he might make it worse by movement), his behaviour (elastic bandage and keeping it still) and his previous experience (what had helped his previous knee injury) that led to his symptoms being prolonged despite his best intentions to make his elbow better. This complicated interaction happens in many situations. Often it is very difficult to reverse this process once it has started.

Uncertainty certainly made John's situation worse – he was not sure what was wrong, what was best to do about it and was not sure that his doctor was making the right decisions. This could maybe have been avoided with a much clearer explanation at the start but the doctor did not know about John's beliefs and so could not predict what would happen. Fortunately, having a friend who had benefited from physiotherapy helped John to be more willing to try this option even though he was not really convinced it would help.

Uncertainty can be based around three main questions:

1 The **cause** of the symptoms.

2 **What can be done** about the symptoms.

3 What will happen in the **future**.

Everyone develops their own sets of beliefs about symptoms and their possible cause. Often, what people think will be influenced by their previous personal experience (such as illnesses in the past) and also those of the people they know. It will depend on how much you know about how your body works and what you might have read in books and papers, on the internet or seen on TV. Doctors will often tell you what you *haven't* got but sometimes are less clear on what you *have* got.

Most people feel uncomfortable with uncertainty and will try to seek definite answers. Clear explanation from doctors may help with this but sometimes they cannot give us all the answers we need and we are left uncertain. Time often allows this uncertainty to reduce. If your symptoms go on for a long time you tend to get used to them and begin to know more about how they affect you: what makes them better, worse, the things you are unable to do, to predict the nature of your attacks, etc. People learn how different situations affect them and naturally tend to avoid things that seem to make them worse and choose things that seem more helpful – we become our own expert for our own symptoms.

This helps predict what might happen to someone in day-to-day life and also helps to manage their symptoms. However, sometimes this can be less helpful than it would first appear. If a person is ill for a long time, they can narrow down their options of what they think and do. This may make them less likely to try alternatives which may actually help. In some situations, through their best intentions, people might even make the situation worse. For example, sometimes symptoms can be prolonged by what you do even though you think you are doing things for the best.

Another common way to reduce uncertainty about illness is to see all the symptoms as part of the same illness. This is a very natural thing to do but may stop you from finding an explanation that allows other things to also be present. Often there are many factors involved, and these may even overlap. The earlier sections in this workbook have shown just how complicated these body processes can be and also how much they can link together. Sometimes it may be easier to tackle symptoms if you can find a way to tease them apart and change the way you view your situation. The rehabilitation approach of this manual aims to provide ways to do this and you can read more about how this works in the next section.

SECTION 5: Medicine and other treatments

Why medicines are used

Most of us will have tried some form of medicine to treat their symptoms at some stage. This might be over the counter, from their GP or recommended by the hospital specialists. This section aims to discuss the most common treatments in a little bit more detail. It will not, however, describe individual medicines as questions on specific medicines are best discussed with the doctor who prescribes them.

There are lots of medicines that have effects on our nervous system and they can be loosely grouped into different types. The main groups are listed below in more detail. The thing they all have in common is that they can affect the transmission of messages around the nervous system. As described earlier in this workbook, messages are passed between one nerve and the next by special chemicals or 'neurotransmitters'. Some of these medicines directly affect the neurotransmitters and others work by methods that are not yet clear.

Some of their effects will overlap, so different groups of medicines may be used to treat exactly the same symptoms. This allows doctors a choice of what to prescribe for different people. And it may be that one person has to try a series of different types before they find one that suits them.

More confusingly, the same medicine may be used in many different clinical situations. Consider, for a moment, a very common medicine that most people are familiar with: aspirin.

Aspirin has always been used to treat pain or for fever, but in recent years it has also been prescribed to protect people after a heart attack or certain types of stroke. In the same way, 'anti-depressants' can be used in many situations that are not depression and 'anti-epileptic' medicines are used by many people who do not have epilepsy. The group names can be confusing because these are based on the first things that these drugs were used for, so anti-depressants may also be used for treatment of pain (including the phantom limb pain you read about earlier) and for many other neurological symptoms, and the same is true of the anti-epileptics.

Common medicines

Benzodiazepines – such as diazepam

This group of medicines has been mainly used as relaxants, either for the muscles or the nervous system. They can treat muscle spasm, make you feel less anxious or help you to sleep. They can also be used for epileptic seizures.

They can be very useful in the short term but, unfortunately, if taken over a longer time the body can become used to them and so they seem to become less effective. Sometimes people end up using bigger and bigger doses to get the same effect. Because of this doctors don't like to prescribe these benzodiazepines for long periods but may suggest them for a short term or intermittent treatment. If, however, someone has been taking them for a long time, it is important that they don't stop them suddenly but reduce the dose gradually with their doctor's supervision. These medicines can have extra side effects if mixed with alcohol, so this combination is best avoided.

Beta-blockers such as propranolol

This group of medicines was originally used to treat people with heart problems such as angina, for protection after heart attacks and for high blood pressure. They can also be used for people with migraine, for thyrotoxicosis (too much of the hormone produced by the thyroid gland) and may be used when people have physical symptoms of anxiety or panic. They have many effects all around the body but can usefully reduce the heart rate and blood pressure.

As we have already mentioned, both these increase at times of stress and, because you can notice your heart beating faster, this can add to the cycle. By preventing this normal response you can break this cycle. Beta-blockers are not addictive and can be used either regularly or just when they are needed. Certain conditions, such as asthma, can be made worse by these medicines so it is important to only take them under prescription from your own doctor.

Anti-depressants

There are several groups of anti-depressants and a great many different medicines within those groups which we will not describe in detail here. As mentioned above, while still called 'anti-depressants' they are often used in many other situations that are not caused by depression. In particular they can be used for pain, especially neuropathic pain (which is thought to come from heightened sensitivity in the nerves) and other chronic pain, and sometimes for reducing functional neurological symptoms. Some can also be used to reduce feelings of anxiety and panic. The way they work is complex and may not be by the same action that they treat depression.

The two main groups you might have come across are the tricyclic anti-depressants (such as amitriptyline or imipramine) and the SSRI (selective serotonin reuptake inhibitor) group (such as fluoxetine or citalopram). There are some differences between these anti-depressants, so people may find one works better or has fewer side effects for them than another.

In general, the tricyclic group has been found to be more effective in people with functional neurological symptoms. Often any side effects will be more noticeable for the first few weeks and then become less bothersome. The useful effects, however, do the opposite as they take time to begin working (usually around two weeks) and can take up to six weeks or more to have their best effect. This may lead people to give up this type of treatment before it has really had time to work.

There is a lot of debate in the press about whether or not anti-depressants are addictive and this sometimes puts some people off trying them. A few people have noticed new symptoms that develop temporarily when stopping their anti-depressant treatment. This is known as 'discontinuation syndrome'. However, if they are stopped gradually there are usually no problems with finishing treatment and these medicines are not addictive.

Research has shown that you are three and a half times more likely to get better from functional symptoms on anti-depressants than without them. This is true whether you are depressed or not. There is also very good evidence that tricyclic anti-depressants are a helpful treatment for people with chronic pain. Further detail about individual anti-depressants and their effects and side effects is beyond the scope of this workbook, but if you have any concerns or questions talk to your doctor.

Anti-epileptic medicine such as gabapentin

This group of medicines was initially used for the treatment of epileptic seizures but is now also used for a variety of neurological symptoms including pain and functional symptoms. It is not clear how these medicines work but they are often tried for prolonged symptoms, particularly if the anti-depressant group has not been tolerated. You don't need to stop driving just because you are taking anti-epileptic medicines.

Painkillers

There are a number of different types of painkillers or 'analgesics' that can be bought over the counter and also prescribed by doctors. Most people will find that they tend to take the one that suits them best and treat themselves on a regular or intermittent basis with over-the-counter painkillers. The main ones include paracetamol, aspirin and the anti-inflammatory drugs such as ibuprofen. Sometimes there might be caffeine or codeine added to these medicines to boost the pain-relieving effects.

There are also stronger prescription painkillers, which include opiate-based medicines and specific treatments for migraine. Unfortunately, prolonged use of opiates may lead to dependency and addictions. Sometimes a combination of different types may be used to control severe pain but in most cases it is sufficient to take just one medicine at a time. Some pain does not respond to painkillers and can even be made worse by people's well-intentioned attempts to treat it. In general, painkillers may be helpful if used for a brief period but they are not a good long-term solution. Finding other ways of coping can often be the answer. Later we describe a problem called rebound headache which can be caused by painkiller use.

The pros and cons of taking medicine

No medicine is without side effects at all. Often it is a balance of what best suits an individual. If there is a noticeable improvement in symptoms some people are willing to put up with more side effects. In general, medicines can be helpful but are usually not the whole solution.

Practical problems taking medicine

Starting

Many patients with functional neurological symptoms find they have a heightened sensitivity to medicines. This leads to greater side effects than would be expected in the general population and often treatment has to be started at a lower dose than usual. A slow increase in dose can also be helpful.

Setting a routine, and forgetting

It is sometimes very difficult to remember to take medicine on a regular basis. This is even worse if someone is taking several different medicines or taking them a number of times throughout the day. Everyone has had the experience of starting a course of antibiotics and doing well at the start but as the week goes on and they improve, they often begin to miss doses or even forget if they have taken them or not. For this very reason, many modern drugs are designed to be taken just once a day. Unfortunately some of the medicines we have described work best if they are given at regular intervals throughout the day.

> KEY POINT
>
> **It is important to find a method that works for you so that you can get the maximum benefit from your treatment.**

Generally people find taking their medicine at a regular time every day helps. Sometimes people use a reminder such as a note on their fridge door, or even a chart to tick off when they have taken it. They may count out the day's medicine in the morning and put it somewhere separate to the main bottle to keep track of how many they have had, or even, if a lot of medicines are involved, use some form of weekly dosette box to simplify the task. You can buy such boxes (which have daily compartments to help you remember when to take tablets) from your local chemist.

Not following the prescription

This is a very common problem which is easy to do. Often people initially take their medicine exactly as their doctor prescribed it and then, as they get used to both their symptoms and their treatment, they might begin to take it differently. This might be:

- More often than prescribed.
- In different situations than prescribed.
- The temptation to use other people's medicines yourself.

In some cases this may be actually harmful, for example taking too much paracetamol may cause liver damage. In others, while not dangerous, it may not add any benefit and so will just increase the risk of side effects without any useful effect. Sometimes it might be that the effects of the medicine have reduced and a change might be helpful. If you find yourself wanting to take your medicine differently it is best to discuss this with your doctor.

Analgesia-induced headache

This is a very specific problem which can occur through the use of regular painkillers. People with frequent headaches tend to take painkillers to either treat or prevent their headaches. Unfortunately, it seems that the use of the painkillers themselves can actually cause more headaches and so a vicious circle of analgesia and *rebound headache* can occur. It is thought that about 20 per cent of patients with chronic headaches and most people with daily headaches have analgesic-rebound headaches.

The mechanism for this is not clear but stopping the use of painkillers for a period can in many cases cure the headaches. These headaches can happen when the painkillers are used frequently for a pain somewhere else in the body too. Again, if you have worries about this you might like to ask your doctor about it.

Other treatments

Medicine is, of course, only part of the treatment for the symptoms discussed in this workbook. Other approaches will be mentioned in later workbooks and include:

- Cognitive Behavioural Therapy (CBT).
- Relaxation and breathing techniques.
- Pacing things so you make changes one step at a time.

- Graded exercise by building exercise slowly and with a plan.
- Physiotherapy.
- Acupuncture.

At this stage it is helpful to consider your current goal. If you think that hyperventilation may be making your symptoms worse you might like to find out more about breathing exercises (in Toolbox D). If you think that relaxation techniques might help you, these can also be found in Toolbox D. Or you may just like to move on to the next workbook.

My current goal

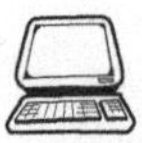

You can get additional help and support in problem solving at www.livinglifetothefull.com

Acknowledgements

The use of the Five Areas assessment model and associated language is used from the Overcoming Five Areas series by permission of Hodder Arnold Publishers and Dr C Williams. Illustrations are by Keith Chan and are reproduced with permission.

My notes

Part 2
Making changes

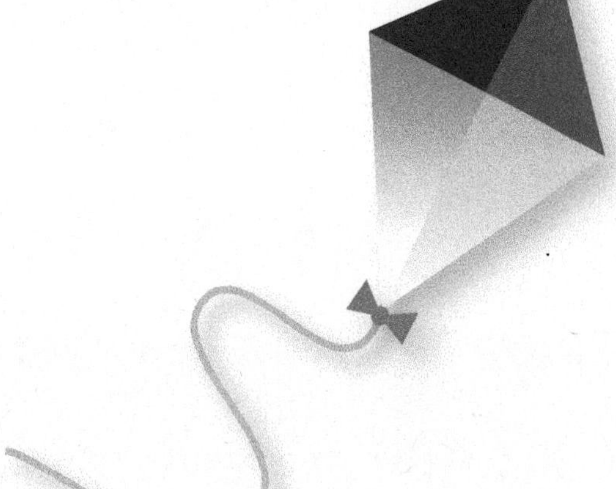

Workbook 3

Five Areas Approach to improving things

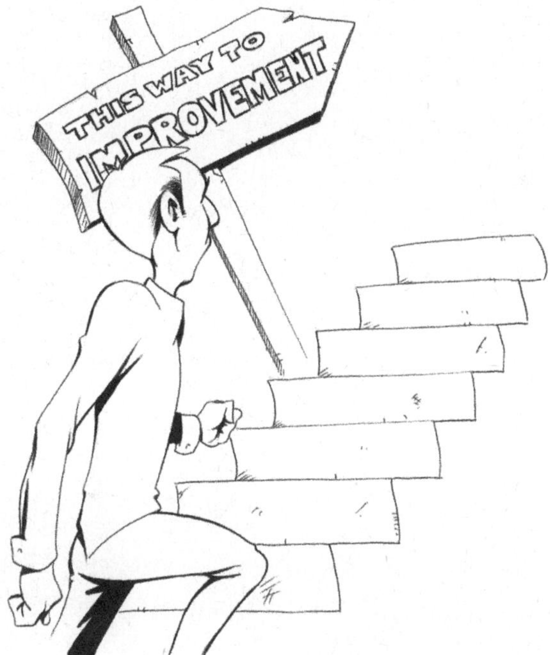

overcoming
functional neurological symptoms:
A Five Areas Approach

SECTION 1: Introduction

Workbook 1 gave a brief introduction to the Five Areas Approach and the links between people's symptoms, thoughts, feelings, behaviour and situation. Sometimes it might be difficult to see how these different areas might affect your symptoms. In particular, can changing how you think and behave actually have an effect on your feelings and symptoms?

Symptoms happen all the time but the more aware people become of them, the more they notice them. Most people will get headaches from time to time. Mostly these are nothing to worry about but sometimes people can think that they might be due to a brain tumour or an impending stroke, if they persist beyond 'normal'. You may never think about the tip of your little finger until you get a paper cut, then you are aware of it all the time. And almost everyone has experienced that when a problem affects your gums or teeth, it is impossible to keep your tongue away.

People's experiences affect how they think about their symptoms. If a relative has had a heart attack then you might naturally worry that twinges of chest pain may be a heart attack too. If you know someone with multiple sclerosis (MS) then any symptoms you have that overlap with them may make you worry you have MS.

In this workbook you will learn about:

- **How thoughts and symptoms affect each other.**
- **How paying attention to symptoms or body processes alters how they feel.**
- **How worry and stress can affect how you feel.**
- **The impact of activity on your symptoms.**
- **Helpful and unhelpful responses you can do.**

The next sections will show how these areas link together.

SECTION 2: How thoughts and symptoms affect each other

The spotlight of the mind – the thought/symptom link

One of the ways that your mind can influence how you react to symptoms depends upon the extent to which your mind is focused on them. This is described as the *spotlight of the mind.* Where this spotlight is focused affects the things you are most aware of.

Think about a time when you may been engrossed in a sport or an activity? You may have fallen over and scuffed a knee but continued playing. After the game you suddenly realised that you have been bleeding. It is only then that you notice the pain. In this example, the spotlight of the mind was originally focused on the excitement of the game. Although the knee has been injured all this time, the pain is only noticed when the game ends.

> KEY POINT
> **The spotlight of the mind can have a large impact on your symptoms.**

If your focus is mainly on your symptoms, they will preoccupy your thoughts and worsen how you feel. Paying attention to symptoms can sometimes cause them to build up and up. Finding other things that you can become interested, occupied or active in can be a big help in coping with long-term symptoms.

Experiment

To see if this process might affect your own experience, try the following experiment. Choose one of your symptoms.

1 On the scale below, rate how much you notice your symptom **now**.

Not present at all										**The worst it's ever been**
0	1	2	3	4	5	6	7	8	9	10

2 Now, focus on your symptom. Consider how you feel, and if it is affecting you. Do this for a short time and then again record how much you notice it.

Not present at all										**The worst it's ever been**
0	1	2	3	4	5	6	7	8	9	10

3 Ask a friend or family member to notice a time when you are engrossed in something, for example watching your favourite soap, talking to someone or reading a book, and then repeat the rating then.

Not present at all										**The worst it's ever been**
0	1	2	3	4	5	6	7	8	9	10

Review: Having done this, what impact does paying attention to your symptoms (2), and being engrossed in other things (3) have on you?

Write your conclusions here:

You may find that that there is no impact, in which case the spotlight of the mind may not be relevant to you.

If you found that the rating worsened at all when you paid attention to it, or reduced at all when you were engrossed, then this is very useful information. It means that your focus on the symptoms may play a part in how you feel. This gives you a possible area to work on as you consider ways of moving forwards.

Paying attention to symptoms or body processes alters how they feel

A second aspect of the spotlight of the mind is that when you pay attention to something it can begin to feel different/strange. To illustrate this, imagine you are in a conversation when someone mentions head lice or nits. As you talk to them, do you notice any difference in how your own scalp feels. You may have become itchy. If you then scratch that area, the itching often then spreads around your scalp. You may notice that other parts of your body also start to feel itchy and uncomfortable.

To find out whether this same process does affect you, try the following experiments.

Experiment

Experiment 1: At rest, pay attention to your breathing for several minutes. Think in detail about the whole process of breathing – especially how much you breathe in and out. Think about how this process seems to work.

Experiment 2: As you walk around, start thinking about how you walk. For example, which joints are moving and how the muscles are working. Think about how you keep balanced and stable as you do this.

Write what you notice here:

Q Does paying attention to your body alter how it feels? Yes ☐ No ☐

Q If **Yes**: does it feel normal or begin to feel abnormal/odd in any way?

Normal ☐ Abnormal/odd ☐

KEY POINT

Sometimes paying attention to quite normal everyday bodily functions makes them seem a little odd or different from usual.

How people view things – the thought–feeling link

Have you ever watched an Olympic boat race or any similar sporting event where there are two fiercely competitive teams? In this race there are two super-fit crews. Each crew puts all their efforts into propelling their boat to victory. Imagine it is one of those years where the boats are neck and neck as they approach the finishing line. As they cross it, one boat just inches ahead and wins. As the cameras focus in on the winning team they are jubilant.

In contrast, the losing crew looks very different. They are silent and dejected, breathing heavily and slumped into their boat. They feel the agony in their arms and legs caused by their exertions. Yet, if it was suddenly announced that the first boat was being disqualified, there would be a rapid change in people in the second boat. They would be thrilled. Their focus on their tired bodies would quickly disappear.

This short description illustrates an important point. How you interpret things can have a marked impact on how you feel. The difference can be dramatic, as shown above. Although this is an extreme example, there is something useful to be learned. In times of illness, people are sometimes very aware of symptoms such as pain, or tiredness or sickness. How you interpret and make sense of these will affect how you feel. It will affect whether you feel calm and peaceful or depressed, angry, worried or ground down.

KEY POINT

This connection between feelings and thoughts can also link to how you experience your symptoms.

SECTION 3: Worry, stress and symptoms

Worries and stress about symptoms can strongly affect how people feel. Sometimes you can focus on illness and mistake everyday symptoms as being caused by serious illness. For example, someone like Patrick (see p. 83) who has heart disease may focus on normal variations in his heart rate. He becomes scared of doing things that raise his heart rate just in case it is dangerous. These fears prevent him going out for walks as recommended by his doctor. It raises the possibility that people can sometimes be overly protective of themselves. To make a decision about the **right balance** of activity you need to seek clear advice from doctors and healthcare practitioners that is based on their professional assessment of your current symptoms. Problems arise when people either ignore this and overdo things, or become overly aware of illness and avoid doing anything at all.

How does this situation arise?

Have you changed where you live recently or do you know of anyone who has? Think about that experience. As someone looks to buy or rent a flat or house, they suddenly begin to notice that there are a lot of houses advertised wherever they go. Similarly when someone changes their car they find that everyone is now driving the same model! The key point here is that you become very aware of things that are relevent to you at the time. This also applies to symptoms and health-related information. When people are worried about symptoms and their consequences, they tend to watch out for information that is relevent to them. This especially applies to anything that might be threatening or scary.

For example, if you have rheumatoid arthritis, you are more likely to pay attention to newspaper or television reports about new treatments of this disease. The same principle applies to how you scan and pay attention to symptoms that seem particularly threatening.

These responses occur in everyone. For example:

- Large screening programmes by occupational health departments often pick up possible problems such as high blood pressure (hypertension) or abnormal ECG (electrocardiogram) heart tracing results. Those people are then referred on for a specialist assessment 'just to be sure'. Most of those people are then given a clean bill of health. Despite this, some of these people will have concerns about their heart that they didn't have before. The health 'scare' has upset them. Even though they are not ill, they feel worse than before.

- Medical students often visit the doctor with health concerns about the area of health that they are studying at the time. For example, they are more prone to present with bowel symptoms shortly after learning about all the different diseases that affect the bowel.

The two examples show how common health anxieties are. These health fears usually fall away quite quickly over a period of weeks or months but sometimes they persist. This is called **health anxiety**.

Health anxiety

In health anxiety, worrying thoughts are focused upon fears about health. A person will feel ill, and believe that they have a potentially dangerous disease. Because what you think affects how you feel emotionally and physically, you feel anxious and notice a number of the physical symptoms of anxiety. Because what you believe also affects what you do, you understandably go to see the doctor.

These reactions are all very similar to a normal response to illness. The key difference here is that there is either no disease present, or the extent of disease cannot explain why the person feels so ill. In spite of normal physical investigations and tests, they may not be reassured. Reassurance in fact just makes things worse. They go again and again to the doctor and are often referred on to other healthcare practitioners for further reassurance. Throughout this the person continues to feel ill.

Patrick's story

After a mild heart attack, Patrick becomes convinced that his heart is not working properly. As a result he constantly feels anxious and is preoccupied with his illness. He feels physically tense and cannot sleep. He is overly aware of any sensations of tension in his chest, and of his heart rate. He keeps checking his pulse rate using a stopwatch. Every time he notices his heart speeding up he is even more convinced that he is seriously ill in spite of 'all-clear' investigations by his specialist.

Patrick is now repeatedly arranging to see his general practitioner (GP) and asking for more tests. He has stopped any activities that he fears may bring on a heart attack, such as doing exercise. This has led to arguments with his wife that have further added to his problems. Exercise has been recommended as part of his rehabilitation programme and should be perfectly safe.

Both Naz in Workbook 2 and Patrick in this example developed excessive worry and stress, which added to their current difficulties.

SECTION 4: Symptoms and your behaviour/activity levels

The impact of activity on your symptoms

Although it can sometimes seem that 'Nothing I do makes any difference', this may not be the case. How you feel can be affected by all sorts of different things you do throughout the day. These changes may seem so subtle that at first you are not even aware of them. To find out what life factors affect how you feel, you might like to try this experiment.

Experiment

Create a diary for **one day** using the blank ones in the Toolbox on pages 211 to 214. Every hour record what you are doing and the severity of your symptoms on a regular basis. Use this to find out what factors might have a similar impact in your own life.

The diary records:

The *time* of day

What you are doing. This might include things like lying in bed listening to the radio; washing the dishes; talking to the boss; sitting in the chair; talking to someone on the phone, having a bath, etc.

Also, record the intensity of your main symptom. You may have a number of different symptoms. Choose to monitor just **one** main symptom (e.g. tingling, weakness, breathlessness, pain, tiredness, stiffness) and record the intensity of this key symptom at this time. Use a scale where 0 means not present at all, and 10 means the worst it has ever been. A score of 5/10 records a moderately severe level.

It's important to only complete the diary for an average day, it can be unhelpful to focus on symptoms in this way over a longer period of time.

Example

Patrick is noticing chest pain throughout the day. He records his symptoms of chest pain on an hourly basis. He uses a watch with an hourly bleep on it as a reminder to fill in the diary. The following is part of his diary where he records his symptoms of chest pain.

Time	What am I doing at the moment?	Intensity of the main symptom (0-10)
9 am	Getting up and having a shower	0/10
10 am	Opening the gas bill, which is higher than expected	7/10
11 am	Talking to personnel on the phone about returning to work	9/10
12 pm	Talking to my wife about our holiday plans for next year	3/10.
1 pm	Going to see my doctor about the investigations.	5/10 before going in to see her. Rising to 7/10 as we talked about the results and she took my blood pressure
2 pm	Listening to the match on the radio.	2/10. It was a good match. We won!
3 pm	Going for a walk with my wife	2/10 to start with increasing to 6/10 when we walked faster than I felt comfortable with.

You can see from his diary that Patrick has discovered something important. His chest pain is not unchanging throughout the day. Instead he feels better when he is taking a shower, talking to his wife about nice things such as holidays, and engrossed in following his favourite team. In contrast, it worsens when he is talking about the symptoms to his doctor, dealing with stressful events such as the gas bill and talking to personnel, and when he walks faster than he feels comfortable with.

Patrick notices:

- Learning to relax and planning in times to wind down may help the pain.
- Anxiety may worsen the symptoms.
- Physical exercise may worsen the symptoms. For example, angina may cause chest pain when he exercises. Specific investigations and advice from his doctor would be needed to find out if this is the case.

The diary therefore provides Patrick with some clear ideas that he can try out. For example, he could build in some time to relax each day during a bath or shower. He could also learn ways to challenge his worries that arise when he thinks about bills and returning to work. He should arrange to see his doctor to see if his chest pain is caused by a physical problem such as angina. In the meantime he should continue to walk at a pace he can cope with and not stop exercising completely.

More on the behaviour/symptom link

Excessive awareness/checking for illness

You have already discovered that becoming overly aware of specific physical symptoms can bring them into the spotlight of the mind. When people notice symptoms, they also try to monitor them. This is especially true of symptoms that you are scared of. So, for example, if you find a lump, you may keep touching it or checking its size in case it gets larger. However, this checking can also **create** symptoms if it is excessive.

Experiment 1

Examine your own forearm and see if you can find a lumpy piece of muscle. Tap this gently with your hand for a minute. Now compare that area with the same area on the other arm.

Q Does the lump feel the same as before? Yes ☐ No ☐

Q Has it altered in size? Yes ☐ No ☐

Q Does it feel the same as your other arm? Yes ☐ No ☐

Q *What is the worst-case scenario that could explain a lump that has increased in size/feels hotter/more painful, etc.?*

KEY POINT

After touching it repeatedly, it is likely that the 'lump' now feels bigger, more tender, and may be more sensitive. The same impact would occur if you repeatedly checked any lump over a number of days or weeks. Checking can make you more aware of the symptom, and actually worsens it.

Experiment 2

Sometimes people become concerned that they have a problem with their throat. It is quite understandable to therefore check how your throat looks and to be especially aware of any sensations there. You might do this by looking into the mirror and saying 'Aaah'. You may also check your throat by swallowing. Let's try an experiment. What happens if you swallow again and again? Take four large swallows one after another to find out.

Q Does your swallowing seem easy? Does it become difficult swallowing? Write what you notice here:

Q What is the worst possible explanation that can explain these symptoms – e.g. that swallowing is becoming difficult?

Of course, sometimes lumps are caused by cancer, and all sorts of throat problems can occur. However, sometimes paying extra attention to an area of the body can start to create or worsen symptoms.

Although you need to keep an eye on your body, for example by regular self-examination of your breasts or testicles, it is the extent of this checking that can become inappropriate. Constantly checking your body not only focuses unhelpfully on symptoms, but in fact the checking itself can begin to create or worsen symptoms.

Checking behaviour can include a wide range of things such as measuring your temperature or blood pressure again and again. The problem isn't doing this just once or twice. It is the excessive focus on the checking that becomes part of the problem. It doesn't reassure you, and indeed reinforces any underlying health fears.

KEY POINT

Sometimes checking behaviour can worsen how you feel.

Write down any excessive checking behaviour here:

Reassurance seeking from others again and again

At one extreme a person may choose not to talk at all about how ill they feel. Keeping problems to yourself may be because you believe 'it is a sign of weakness to be ill or to be seen as not coping'. At the other extreme, another person may recurrently seek support and *excessive reassurance* again and again from others. This is again a good example of an action that in moderation can be *helpful*, but which can become *unhelpful* when taken to excess. The result is a feeling of dependency on others and a further loss of confidence in yourself.

> **KEY POINT**
> **The more reassurance a person gets, the more they seek it.**

Excessive self-medication

When you are ill, you are often prescribed medication to treat the disorder. It can be tempting sometimes to take an extra dose of tablet if you feel worse at a particular time. This raises the possibility of taking too high a dose. The danger is of serious side effects. For example, some medications prescribed for pain can lead to kidney or liver problems if taken for too long or at too high a dose. Tablets should always therefore be taken as indicated on the prescription and the dose reviewed with your doctor from time to time.

Pushing others away or becoming angry about your symptoms

Another natural but unhelpful reaction is resolving feelings by turning against those around you. People may become angry, gossipy and undermine others by spreading rumours or become bitter and critical. This particularly can occur towards those who are easy targets and less likely to hit back, such as close relatives, your practitioners and friends. Sometimes this behaviour is a form of testing out the love, friendship and support of others. The consequence may be isolation, rejection and loneliness.

Quickly stopping doing activities because of sudden feelings of anxiety or increased symptoms

You can suddenly feel worse for a number of reasons. Sometimes you may have sudden fears that what you are doing will worsen how you feel physically. In Naz's case (see Workbook 2), he has sudden rushes of fear that he will have a stroke. This is where clear medical advice can be really helpful. Anxious fears are often very catastrophic and unrealistic. In Naz's case, these fears are exactly that. He will not bring on a stroke by playing football, but whenever he stops what he is doing and sits down to rest this just confirms to him his belief that it is only by stopping all activity that he is avoiding a stroke.

Filling every moment of your time

Sometimes people unwisely try to fill every part of the day to avoid noticing how ill they feel. This may involve deliberately staying up late watching films, or sleeping in during the day to avoid seeing others. It also could include spending hours on computer games or watching television. Other common activities are listening to music, chatting/surfing on the internet or texting others all the time. This is not to say that such activities are all unhelpful – more about why and how much they are done. Doing these things because they can help avoid life is a very different motivation than doing them because they are fun.

Posture, aids and mobility

When long-term symptoms occur, there is a risk of physical disability. This may have many causes, including the physical disease process and symptoms themselves (for example arthritis or muscular problems such as after a stroke). Long-term reduced activity also can play a part. This leads to muscle weakness and possibly even contractures of underused muscles and joints. Another important factor is that when people have problems such as pain, they alter their posture to attempt to 'protect' painful joints or muscles. There are clear and understandable reasons for this. However, sometimes this attempt to improve things can backfire.

Mirror task

Look at yourself in a full-length mirror. Think about your own posture. Are you holding your own muscles in a very tense way? How balanced and at ease do you seem? If you are, you may be making yourself more prone to muscle strains. This can create or worsen pain symptoms by creating excessive pressures on your back, arms and legs. Similarly, walking with a stick or using a wheelchair can sometimes add to difficulties.

If possible, plan to gradually reduce your use of such aids unless advised otherwise by your healthcare practitioner. Specialist advice is essential here so that if you need any aids, they are the correct ones for you, you know how best to use them and your use of them is reviewed by a healthcare practitioner such as your GP or occupational therapist.

KEY POINT

What can seem helpful in the short term, can become unhelpful in the longer term.

A second problem is that these actions also teach an unhelpful lesson – *that it is only by checking /avoiding or leaving the situation, etc. that you managed to cope*. In the longer term, this behaviour therefore backfires and adds to your problems.

SECTION 5: Helpful and unhelpful behaviours

Helpful and unhelpful behaviours

When people experience symptoms, it is normal to try to do things to feel better. This altered behaviour may be *helpful* or *unhelpful*. The purpose is to help you feel safer/ better – at least in the short term.

Helpful activities may include things you do alone, and things you do with others:

- Talking and receiving support from friends or relatives.
- Reading or using self-help materials so that you and those around you can find out more about the causes and treatment of the problems.
- Maintaining activities that aren't solitary and provide pleasure or support such as meeting friends, attending a class, and attending religious activities.
- Challenging anxious worrying thoughts by stopping, thinking and reflecting rather than accepting them as true.
- Going to see your doctor or healthcare practitioner.

You should aim to try to maximise the number of helpful activities you do as part of your recovery plan. Planning these helpful activities can boost how you feel.

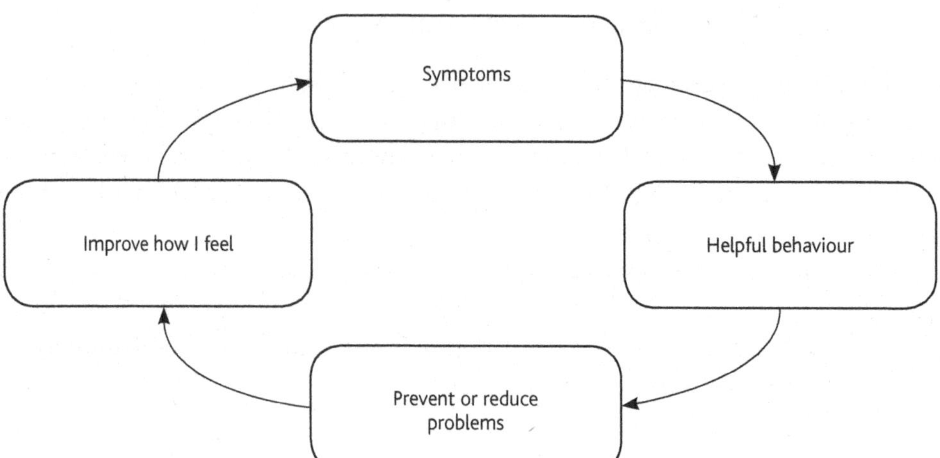

The circle of helpful behaviour.

Checklist: Identifying the circle of helpful behaviour

Am I:	
Being good to myself, e.g. eating regularly and healthily – taking time to enjoy the food?	☐
Keeping as active as I can, e.g. doing exercise/going for walks/swimming/going to a gym?	☐
Stopping, thinking and reflecting on things rather than jumping to conclusions – letting upsetting thoughts 'be' rather than constantly mulling them over?	☐
Pacing myself – and letting others know I am doing this, e.g. telling relatives I am planning to do less, or discussing my needs with occupational health at work. The consequence is others may need to do more and this requires communication to explain why?	☐
Seeing a healthcare practitioner for advice and viewing recovery as an active and joint collaboration. Being honest with them about progress, or when I feel stuck?	☐
Socialising at a level I can cope with – whether that means by telephone, email or going out?	☐
Seeking support from others, e.g. sharing concerns appropriately with trusted friends and family?	☐
Keeping as active as possible when facing situations such as problems with pain. Walking with as much of a relaxed and normal stance as possible?	☐
Using effective coping responses such as relaxation techniques to deal with feelings of tension?	☐
Doing things for fun or pleasure, e.g. hobbies, listening to music?	☐
Doing planned activities at a pace I can cope with?	☐
Taking my prescribed medication regularly and as advised?	☐
Using my sense of humour to cope?	☐

Q *Am I doing any other helpful behaviours?*

Having completed these questions try to build these helpful responses into your life.

KEY POINT

Sometimes you can think that something you are doing is helpful but in the longer term it can become part of the problem.

Unhelpful behaviours

At times, you try to improve how you feel. Unfortunately, you may use a number of *unhelpful behaviours* such as becoming very dependent on others or pushing people away. These actions backfire and create further problems. This can include immediate or longer-term problems, or affect important relationships. These actions therefore act to keep the difficulties going and become part of the problem. A *vicious circle of unhelpful behaviour* may result.

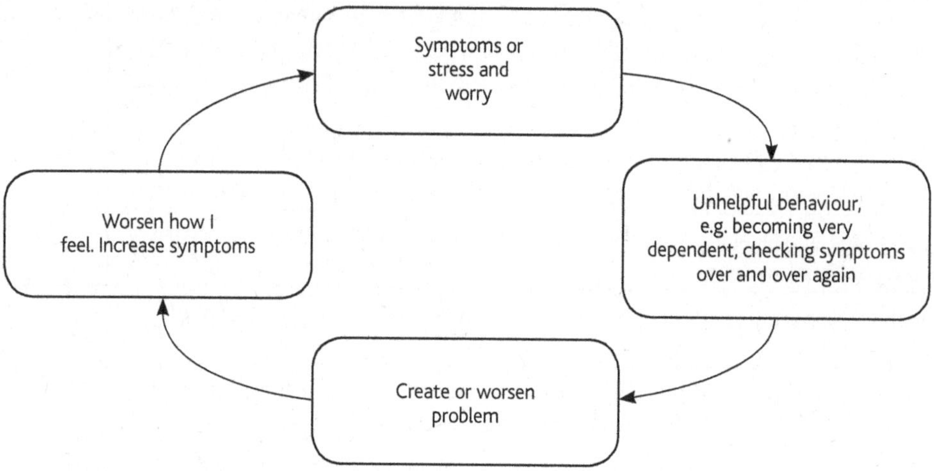

The vicious circle of unhelpful behaviour.

Now take a look at the following list and tick any activity you have found yourself doing in the past few weeks. A wide range of different unhelpful behaviours have been summarised here to help you to think about changes that could be happening in your own life.

Checklist: Identifying the vicious circle of unhelpful behaviour

Am I:	
Throwing myself into doing things so there are no opportunities to stop, think and reflect?	☐
Looking to others to make decisions or sort out problems for me?	☐
Being overly aware and excessive checking for symptoms of ill health?	☐
Becoming very demanding or excessively seeking reassurance from others?	☐
Excessively changing the way I sit or walk to reduce symptoms of physical discomfort? The altered posture then creates or worsens the physical problem.	☐
Pushing others away and being verbally or physically threatening/rude to them?	☐

Taking part in risk-taking actions, for example crossing the road without looking, or gambling using money I don't really have?	☐
Eating too much to block how I feel ('comfort eating'), or over-eating so much that this becomes a 'binge'?	☐
Compulsively checking, cleaning, or doing things a set number of times or in exactly the 'correct' order so as to make things 'right'?	☐
Trying to spend my way out of how I feel by going shopping ('retail therapy')?	☐
Carrying out mental rituals such as counting or deliberately thinking 'good' thoughts/saying prayers to make things feel 'right'?	☐
Deliberately harming myself in an attempt to block how I feel?	☐
Misusing drink/illegal drugs or prescribed medication to block how I feel in general or improve how I sleep, etc?	☐

If you notice such behaviours it can be useful to:

- Plan to slowly reduce any unhelpful behaviours
- While at the same time planning to boost your helpful behaviours

To find out more about how to build helpful behaviours and reduce unhelpful behaviours see Workbooks 3 and 4.

The reactions of others

Sometimes people around you may offer 'helpful advice' all the time and want to do *everything* for you. There can be many reasons for this. Often the cause is concern, friendship and love for you. Sometimes it may be the result of anxiety, or occasionally guilt. Whatever the cause, when others offer too much help and want to do everything for you, their actions can backfire in several ways.

KEY POINT

When trying to cope with symptoms it is important to continue to do as many things as you are able within the confines of how you feel. If others take responsibility for doing everything for you, the danger is that you become less active than you could be.

If this situation seems to be developing for you, Toolbox E may be helpful for those around you to read.

How it all fits together

Let's have another look at Naz and Kate's examples from Workbook 2. How would these fit into the Five Areas Approach?

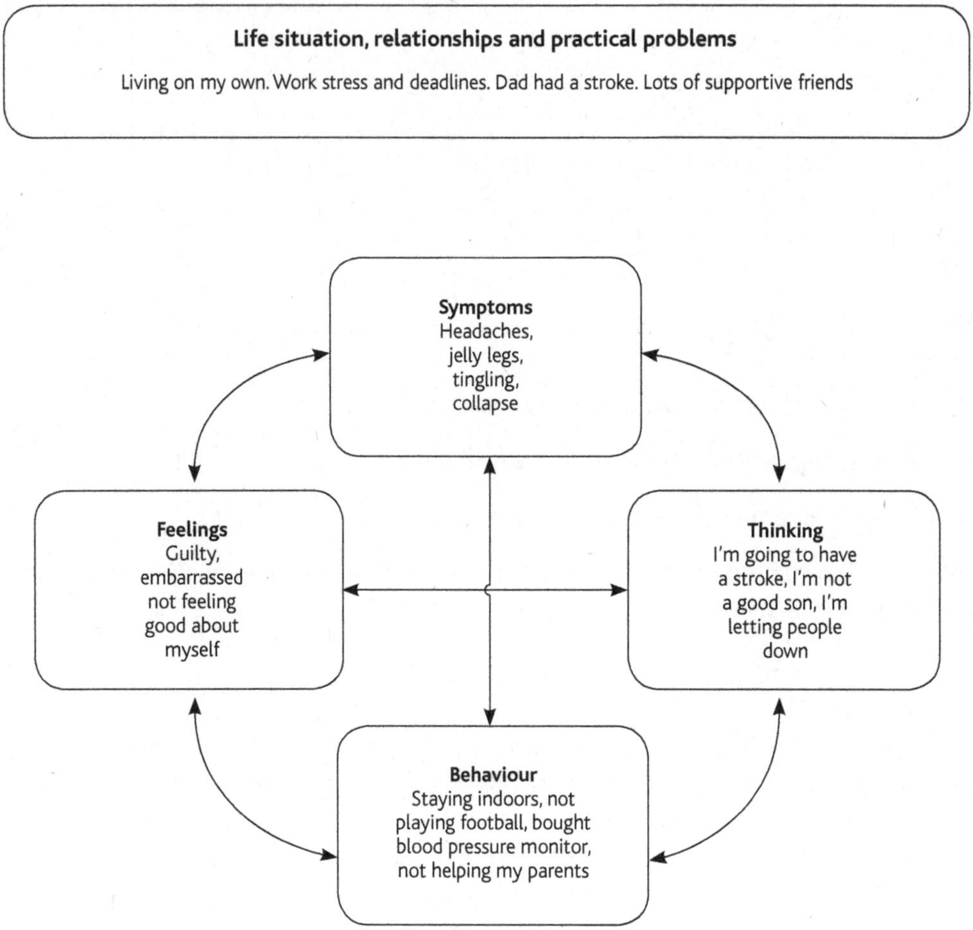

Naz's Five Areas assessment (from Workbook 2, page 34).

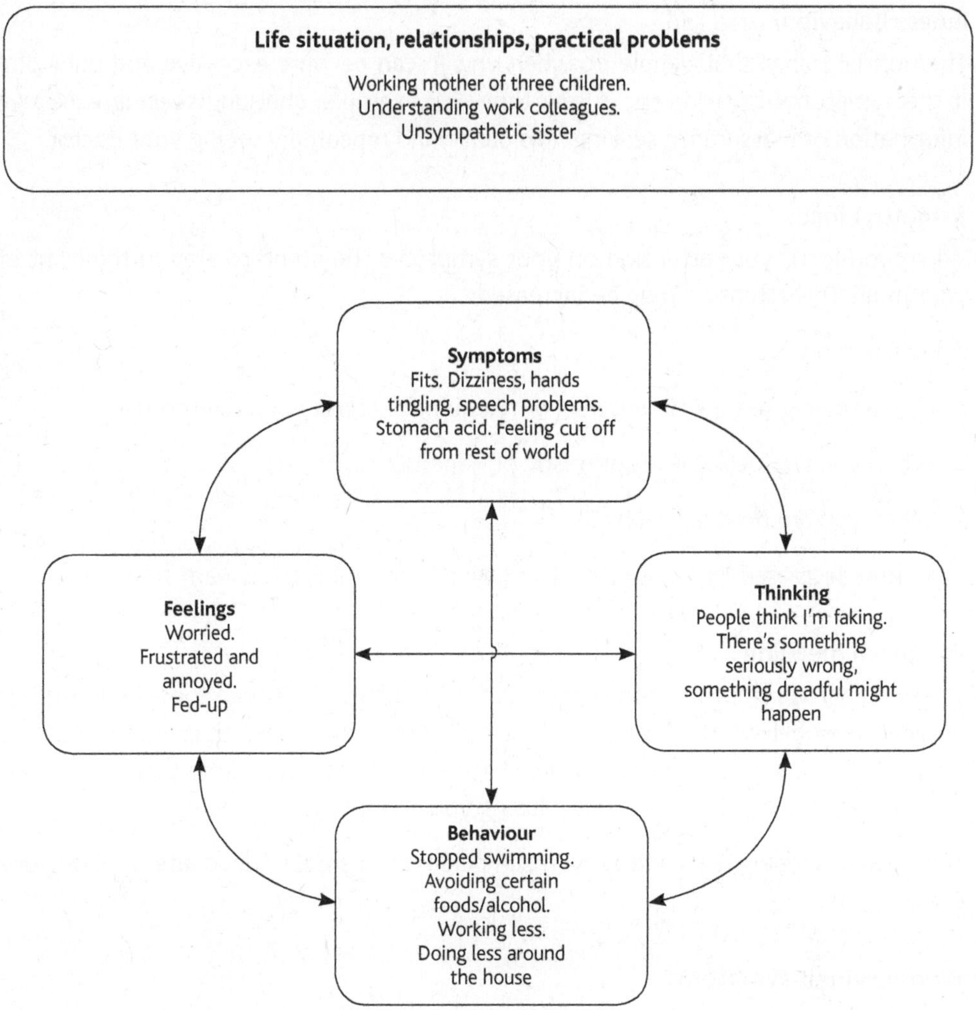

Kate's Five Areas assessment (from Workbook 2, page 35).

As you have just read, making changes in one area can affect the others. Looking at their situations in a different way allows Naz and Kate the opportunity to put this into practice. This is explored in more detail in the later workbooks.

What keeps your symptoms going?

Research has shown that there are many common factors which tend to keep symptoms going no matter how they first started.

Throughout these workbooks you'll come back to these factors again and again. Below we describe the most common ones and where you can find out more about them.

Illness behaviour

The normal things that people do when unwell can become excessive and unhelpful if the symptoms carry on for a long time. For example: checking seeking excessive information or reassurance seeking, avoidance and repeatedly seeing your doctor.

Symptom focus

When you focus your attention on your symptoms they tend to stay in the front of your mind. This attention may be increased:

- By checking.
- By continuing to look for answers or reassurance about your symptoms.
- When you are feeling less optimistic or hopeful.
- When you are tired or feeling ill.

It is often decreased by focusing and engaging in the things you want to do.

Symptom meaning

The exact same symptoms can suggest different things to different people depending on what they believe they mean. For example, you may believe that your symptoms are evidence of something much worse than your doctors have told you or you may misread which part of your body is causing your symptoms.

The ways of keeping fears and concerns in perspective are described later in Workbook 5.

Worries about symptoms

Worry or fear of worsening your situation leads to avoidance or reduced activity. These can be worries about causing further damage, worsening pain or having a setback. Worries that something has been missed or that you may have been given a wrong diagnosis can lead to increased symptom focus.

What can cause more symptoms?

Becoming unfit through lack of exercise and reduced activity can worsen your symptoms. Worries can also make your body's stress system cause more symptoms.

SECTION 6: Summary

In this workbook you have discovered:

- **How thoughts and symptoms affect each other.**
- **How paying attention to symptoms or body processes alters how they feel.**
- **How worry and stress can affect how you feel.**
- **The impact of activity on your symptoms.**
- **Helpful and unhelpful responses you can do.**

Putting what you have learned into practice

Having completed this workbook you should now have a clearer idea of the impact your symptoms are having in all five areas of your life. From your assessment in Workbook 1 you will have identified various target areas to work on. Most people find it easier to start experimenting with their behaviours and this is what you will look at in more detail in the next workbook before turning your attention to thinking. If, however, you feel that you would prefer to start by looking at your thinking then you could move on to Workbook 5. The majority of people find that they notice more improvement when then have worked through both Workbooks 4 and 5 and start putting it all together. To keep you on track it is useful to identify your current goal for your next step. For example, at this stage you may be making a plan to tackle unhelpful behaviours and so using the Toolbox to fill out a diary, or you may be planning to work through Workbook 4.

> **REMEMBER**
> **The workbooks are best used one at a time to learn the techniques. Try not to be tempted to do two at once. By the time you have worked through the whole book it will all fit together. Discuss this with your healthcare practitioner if you are stuck or unsure what to do.**

My current goal

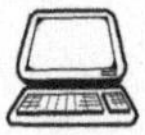

You can get additional help and support in problem solving at www.livinglifetothefull.com

Acknowledgements

The use of the Five Areas assessment model and associated language is used from the Overcoming Five Areas series by permission of Hodder Arnold Publishers and Dr C Williams. Illustrations are by Keith Chan and are reproduced with permission.

My notes

Workbook 4

Behaviours

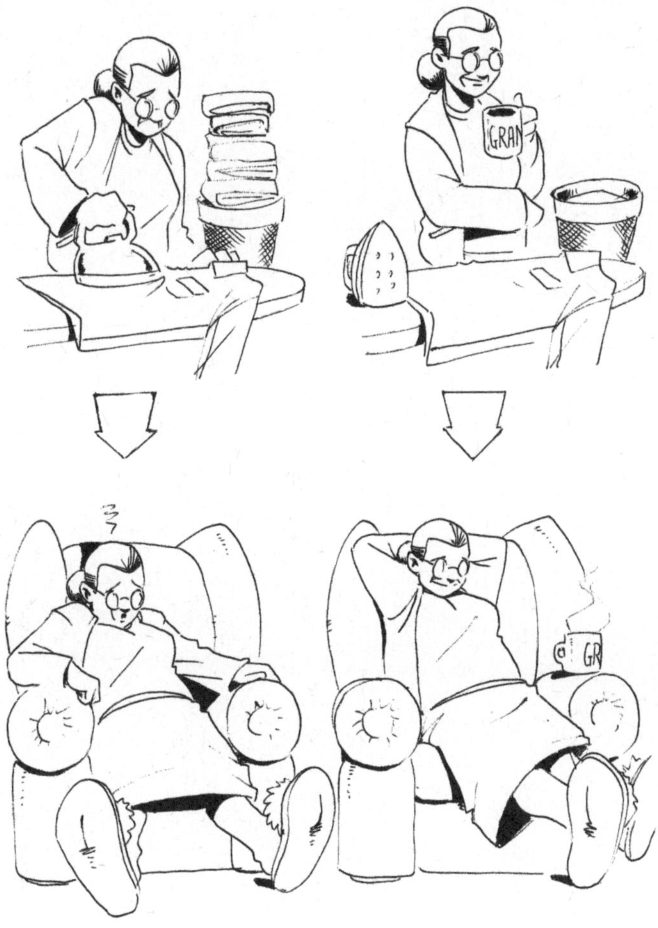

overcoming
functional neurological symptoms:
A Five Areas Approach

SECTION 1: Introduction

Symptoms can often affect your activity levels and restrict what you can do in your life. They can also lead you to avoid, or stop doing, things you used to do. This workbook looks at some practical ways of changing the things you do (your activity levels and behaviours). Although this may seem difficult, the feedback we have had suggests that this workbook can be a very effective way of helping you feel better.

In this workbook you will:

- **Read about examples of people who have found their behaviours have changed in one way or another because of their symptoms.**
  - **David and Kate, who plan a way of increasing their activity levels in order to build activities that they value and actually want to do.**
  - **Jane, who plans ways to overcome her avoidance.**
  - **Naz, who finds a way to challenge his worries about worsening his symptoms.**
- **Learn to identify your own vicious circles of reduced activity or avoidance.**
- **Learn how you can make your own plans for change.**
- **Plan some next steps to keep positive changes going.**

In the past you may have tried all sorts of attempts to change, but unless you have a clear plan and stick to it, change can be difficult. Planning and selecting which changes to try to make first is a crucial part of successfully moving forwards. By choosing which areas to start with, this also means that you are actively choosing at first *not* to focus on other areas.

KEY POINT

Setting targets will help you to focus on how to make the changes needed to get better. To do this you will need:

- ***Short-term* targets: thinking about changes you can make today, tomorrow and the next week.**
- ***Medium-term* targets: changes to be put in place over the next few weeks.**
- ***Long-term* targets: where you want to be in six months or a year.**

The impact of symptoms on your life

The experience of illness affects everyone in unique ways. However, there are three common things which can happen as a result of symptoms:

- A *vicious circle of reduced activity*: When you struggle with symptoms, they often prevent you from doing other things in your life that you enjoy. The result is that important things can become squeezed out. You focus instead on your basic activities such as getting better, looking after children, chores. In other words, the things you feel you must prioritise. This can mean that you are prevented from doing things that previously gave you a sense of pleasure or achievement. For example, you may have stopped going out, meeting up with friends or doing hobbies. By emptying your life of these things you can feel worse as a result.

The good news is that this can be a helpful target area. We will describe how to make such changes in a planned, step-by-step way later in this workbook.

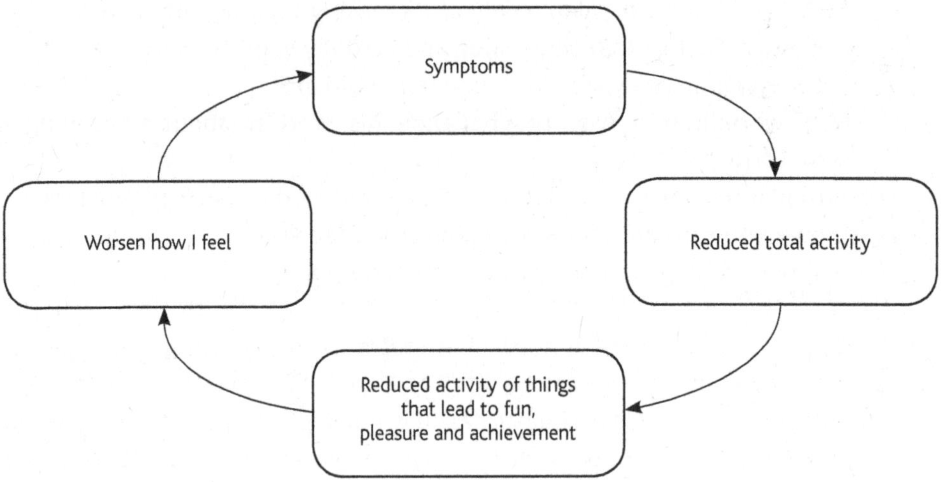

The vicious circle of reduced activity.

- A *vicious circle of unhelpful behaviours*: Symptoms can be both distressing and challenging. How you respond to them can include both helpful and unhelpful reactions. Some unhelpful responses can be obvious, for example taking medication in far higher doses than recommended. Some may be less obvious but still end up backfiring and adding to your problems, such as looking to others to assist you all the time, or becoming irritable or angry and pushing others away. You will find out about this later in this workbook and also about building on helpful responses as well as how to reduce the unhelpful ones.

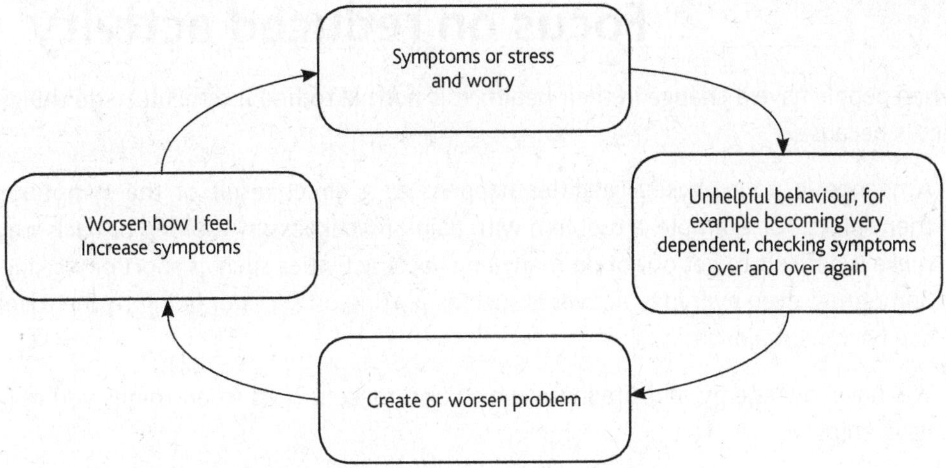

The vicious circle of unhelpful behaviour.

- A *vicious circle of avoidance*. We will look at this more closely later in this workbook.

SECTION 2: Focus on reduced activity

When people have a change in their health, it is normal to find it difficult to do things. This is because:

- A change in your physical abilities happens as a direct result of the symptoms themselves. For example, a problem with pain or weakness in your leg or back may make it difficult to get out or do many enjoyable activities such as sport or walking. Sometimes even everyday activities such as putting on socks or going to the toilet can become major tasks.
- You have low energy and tiredness, which also make it hard to do things you may have enjoyed.
- Worries that you might make your symptoms worse. This is especially the case when pain is one of the symptoms and you may worry that using a painful arm or leg may cause physical damage. Overly reduced activity can lead to increased short-term benefits; however, in the longer term this can result in stiffening of muscles and joints and worsened pain. Instead, slow, steady ways of maintaining and increasing activity can help improve mobility and reduce pain and stiffness.
- When you feel ill a natural response is to rest to allow recovery. Resting can be sometimes helpful, for example to allow acute inflammation to settle. However, there may be some unintended consequences.

Example: Muscle bulk and activity

Unused muscles suffer from a reduction in muscle bulk and they weaken. Research studies with astronauts on the space programme found that they had to carry out regular exercises to use their muscles to prevent muscle wastage while in zero gravity. The same principle applies if you are using your muscles much less often in everyday tasks. Unless you deliberately exercise/use them then muscle wastage will occur.

Rest can also worsen muscle and joint pain – when you rest excessively you tend to stiffen up. This is especially true when staying in one posture such as lying down, sitting in a chair or propping yourself up with multiple pillows for an extended time. Then, when you use the muscles/joints they feel stiff and painful as a result. This is why physiotherapists and doctors advise people to try to maintain activity levels as much as possible.

However, your own thoughts may interfere with whether or not you take this advice. For example:

- Low motivation and reduced enthusiasm to do things ('I just can't be bothered').
- Frustration and little sense of enjoyment or achievement when things are done ('There's no point because I can't do it properly').

A vicious circle of reduced activity may result.

Example: David's story

David is recently retired and has developed pain and weakness in both his legs and now finds it difficult walking far from the house. He also feels fatigued. David was very active before this happened. He really enjoyed going for walks with his wife Anne. He has always been fit and enjoyed sports. He and Anne are no longer able to go for walks together and he is feeling frustrated that he is stuck in the house.

Currently David can walk as far as the car. Anne often drives him to the many hospital appointments he attends. Frustratingly they cannot go shopping. This is something he used to enjoy. He remembers that they would spend a long time chatting to friends as they went from shop to shop. He now finds that for much of the day he sits in his chair watching TV.

Over the months David has found that his legs feel weaker the more he rests. He feels frustrated and angry and is becoming dispirited by the whole situation. He has previously looked down on people who watched daytime TV and is not at all happy that 'things have come to this'.

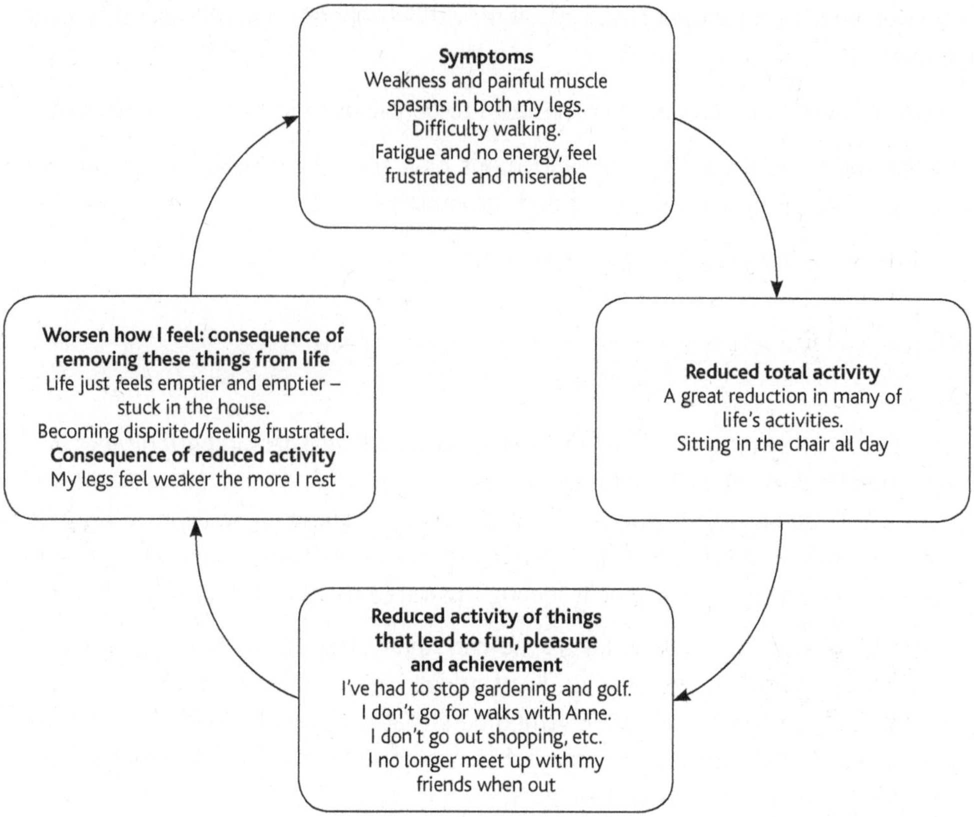

David's vicious circle of reduced activity.

David's first task is to decide whether he has problems of reduced activity that are making him feel worse. He completes a checklist and identifies three areas of reduced activity.

Checklist: David identifies his reduced activity

Reduced or stopped activity or behaviour	*Tick here if you have noticed this*
Noticing symptoms resulting from reduced activity – such as worsened stiffness/pain, restricted joint movement or slowly worsening weakness of under-used muscles	✓ *I stiffen up when I don't get up but my weakness makes it difficult*
Going out/meeting friends	✓ *I have stopped meeting up with my friends*

Reduced or stopped activity or behaviour	*Tick here if you have noticed this*
Neglecting food – eating less or tending to eat more 'junk' food, or food that takes little preparation	✗
Stopping/reducing doing hobbies/interests such as reading or other things you previously enjoyed or did to relax	✓ *I no longer do the garden*
'Letting things go' around the house	✓ *Anne often has to ask me to do odd jobs that I used to do*
Not answering the phone or the door when people visit	✗
Not opening or replying to letters/bills	✗
Other (write in)	

On answering the following questions David determines that he is experiencing a *vicious circle of reduced activity.*

1. Have I stopped doing things I used to enjoy as a result of how I feel?

Yes ✓ No ☐

2. Has the reduced activity:

- Removed things from life that previously gave me a sense of pleasure/achievement?

Yes ✓ No ☐

- Or worsened how I feel physically?

Yes ✓ No ☐

3. Overall, has this worsened how I feel?

Yes ✓ No ☐

Task: Self-review

Think about your own life – there may be areas of reduced activity you have noticed. Complete the checklist now to identify any areas of reduced activities that apply to you.

Checklist: Reduced or stopped activity or behaviour

Am I:	
Going out/meeting friends less than before?	☐

Noticing physical consequences of reduced activity – such as worsened stiffness/pain, restricted joint movement or slowly worsening weakness of under-used muscles?	☐
Neglecting food – eating less or tending to eat more 'junk' food, or food that takes little preparation?	☐
Stopping/reducing doing hobbies/interests such as reading or other things I previously enjoyed or did to relax?	☐
'Letting things go' around the house?	☐
Not answering the phone or the door when people visit?	☐
Not opening or replying to letters/bills?	☐
Other (write in)	

Q 1. Have I stopped doing things I used to enjoy as a result of how I feel?

Yes ☐ No ☐

Q 2. Has the reduced activity

- Removed things from life that previously gave me a sense of pleasure/achievement?

Yes ☐ No ☐

- Or worsened how I feel physically?

Yes ☐ No ☐

Q 3. Overall, has this worsened how I feel?

Yes ☐ No ☐

Choice point

- **If you have answered Yes to at least two of Questions 1–3** then you are experiencing the vicious circle of reduced activity. We suggest you concentrate on the examples of reduced activity in this workbook.
- **If you haven't answered Yes to these questions** it is unlikely that the vicious circle of reduced activity applies to you. You may find the examples of avoidance in Section 2 of this workbook more relevant to you.

Lack of energy and feeling tired

KEY POINT

If fatigue is a problem for you then there are some common myths to bear in mind.

Myth 1: I need to store up my energy for big events

Some people believe that they must store up energy in preparation for demanding situations. If they have a big day coming up such as a family wedding or other event then they rest and do as little as possible for a long period of time before the event. They anticipate that the event will take a lot out of them and so rest beforehand as a precaution. Although this would seem like a logical strategy, this is not how your body most effectively stores and uses energy, and overlay resting will weaken muscles and stop you being active.

Myth 2: Activity runs down my inner resources

Some people are concerned that *any* activity will make fatigue problems worse. They therefore avoid activity, which in the long term actually has the opposite effect of worsening the problem. Inactivity reduces muscle strength and condition and reduces physical fitness. A study of 'healthy' students who were paid to go to bed for several months found that they lost up to 10 per cent of their muscle bulk in the first week of remaining in bed and this deterioration continued. The research also showed that dizziness when standing up, difficulty concentrating/forgetfulness and low mood were common side effects of prolonged bed rest. In addition, change to sudden increase of activity can lead to joint and muscle pain/pulls, etc. However, activity levels can be *slowly increased in a planned way*.

> **REMINDER**
>
> **If you didn't read about how your muscles and joints work together in Workbook 2, it might be helpful to do this now.**

A final common area that needs to be considered is if you are someone who drives/forces themselves to do things – in short, you overdo things.

Overdoing it

Sometimes it can be really tempting to try to return to what you did before feeling ill too quickly. But if you increase your activity too drastically this can have a big impact on your symptoms and on how motivated you feel.

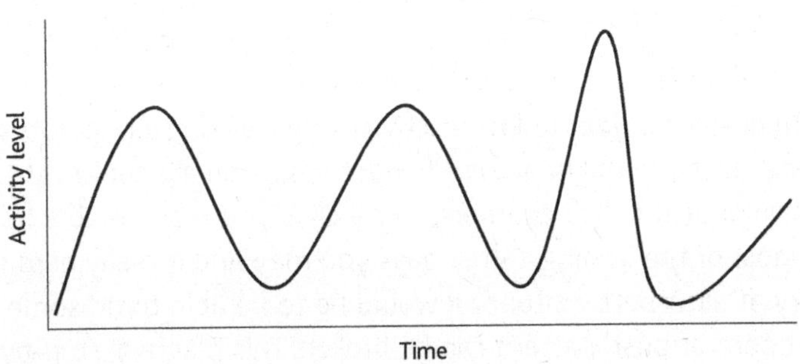

The boom or bust cycle.

For example, if you feel good one day, do you then tend to try to accomplish many outstanding tasks, leaving you exhausted or with worse symptoms for several subsequent days? Or on a 'good day' do you give in to the temptation to be as 'normal' as possible and do as much as you feel you used to? This can also happen when you have a good week and feel almost back to your usual self. Temporarily this may make you feel great but can often lead to a setback. This is known as 'boom or bust' and is quite common, both when you feel at your worst but also when you are recovering.

It can be very frustrating and often seem like one step forwards and two steps back. Sometimes people end up in this cycle because they feel guilty about what those around them have to do for them. In fact, others may expect you to try to do as much as you can when you seem able.

If this applies to you, the most crucial part of the early stage of recovery is to stabilise your activity. One way to start to do this is to record your activity over a week or two using an **activity diary** (see Toolbox, pp. 211 to 214). It is usually helpful to begin with to establish a baseline record of your activities. Often it is easier to do this as you go along rather than trying to remember at the end of the day. It will give you an idea of exactly how active you are at present and also if you are in a 'boom or bust' cycle. Some people are surprised to find patterns emerging of what they do and how it makes them feel.

Example: Recording Caroline's activity

Caroline finds that she can iron for 45 minutes on a good day without stopping. However, on a bad day she can barely manage five minutes. This is summarised below.

	Monday	*Tuesday*	*Wednesday*	*Thursday*	*Friday*	*Saturday*	*Sunday*	*Total*
Time spent	10 min	5 min	45 min	5 min	0 min	0 min	0 min	60 min

Once you have an idea of your current activity levels you can then use the steps to build on this to overcome your reduced activity or pace yourself. For lots of people this will mean that at first you might actually *reduce* what you are currently doing. This can feel very unnatural at first. For example, some days you may be able to do all of the washing and most of the ironing. Other days you may find it really hard to get up and do any laundry at all. A better situation would be to be able to do some every day. In this way the 'boom or bust' pattern can be broken. This planned, step-by-step way of changing your behaviour is known as 'pacing'.

Using the pacing approach

Let's look again at how people can tackle some household chores. You need to find a happy medium between all or nothing. This may mean increasing what you do on bad days but decreasing what you do on good ones. Again this might sound strange and can in practice feel 'wrong'. Another example would be poor concentration stopping you finishing a crossword or reading your newspaper. Again sometimes this might seem easy and other times impossible. It might seem a little strange at first but pacing can help with this too.

You can plan the steps needed to make changes using an **activity plan sheet**, which is included on pages 211 to 214 of the Toolbox.

Example: Caroline's paced approach to her problem

Caroline finds that she can iron for 45 minutes on a good day without stopping. However, on a bad day she can barely manage five minutes. Ideally Caroline should aim between these two levels on both good and bad days. She should aim low and try to do five to 10 minutes every day, no matter whether she feels 'good' or 'bad'. Then she can slowly increase this on a weekly basis. She uses the activity plan sheet to slowly plan the increase in her ironing.

At first Caroline feels she is just not getting enough done and becomes frustrated. However, she soon realises that overall she is actually doing more than she was in her 'boom or bust' cycle. Her plan is summarised below:

Caroline's plan to increase her ironing

New plan	*Monday*	*Tuesday*	*Wednesday*	*Thursday*	*Friday*	*Saturday*	*Sunday*	*Total*
Week 1	5 min	6 min	5 min	7 min	5 min	5 min	5 min	38 min
Week 2	8 min	9 min	9 min	8 min	7 min	8 min	9 min	58 min
Week 3	11 min	12 min	11 min	12 min	11 min	13 min	12 min	82 min
Week 4	14 min	15 min	14 min	15 min	12 min	15 min	15 min	100 min

KEY POINT

The most important thing is to set a plan and stick to it. You need to be consistent and rein yourself in once you have achieved your goal – *even when you feel you could carry on.*

The same principles apply to any activity. It is important to use this same approach for things you value and enjoy as well as chores.

Activity can be defined as anything that stimulates the brain as well as your body. This includes mental activity as well as more physically energetic tasks. Setting a structure which breaks an activity into smaller steps and then 'pacing' them will increase the chances of success. So the idea behind pacing is that the amount that you do is broadly similar on all days and you avoid big peaks and troughs. Your activity levels out, as shown below.

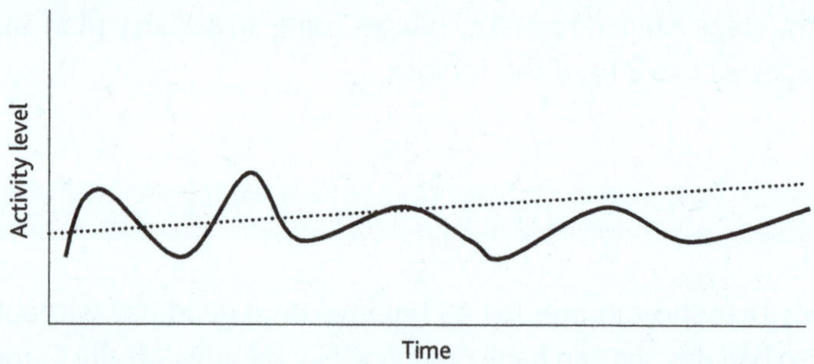

Pacing is the key to slow, step-by-step improvement.

KEY POINT

Pacing can make some people feel frustrated at the start. But most find they improve fairly quickly and benefits are lasting.

SECTION 3: Focus on avoidance

Understanding avoidance

It is natural to try to avoid situations that seem to make you feel worse. If you look at Jane's situation below, you will see that not only has she stopped travelling by bus but she has also stopped socialising with her friends. She has begun avoiding any busy places and now cannot go shopping in the supermarket. She also feels uncomfortable in enclosed spaces. Your own anxiety and worry about what might happen to you can increase your avoidance of certain things. This can happen without you even noticing.

Example: Jane's story

Jane has been referred to the neurology outpatient department by her general practitioner (GP). She didn't really notice when her symptoms first started but things have been getting a lot worse over the past year. She has worked in a sandwich shop for five years and is now the assistant manager.

Jane has a number of symptoms that have started to really affect her life. These are happening more often and in more situations. Jane was with her friends and had a lot of symptoms all at once while in a lift. Her friends were so worried they made her promise to see her GP.

When Jane went to see her GP she described all of her symptoms. Jane feels that her asthma is worse than usual, she often feels unable to take a deep enough breath. She is using her inhaler much more frequently. She told him about her tiredness and vivid dreams which awaken her most nights. Sometimes she lies awake with her heart racing for a long time afterwards. She finds herself yawning all day and by mid afternoon just wants to lie down. Jane has noticed lots of aches around her neck and shoulders and more recently some pains in her chest.

Jane wonders if she has pulled something or whether there is something seriously wrong. More recently she has had tingling in her hands and fingers and numbness in her left arm. Sometimes she even has this around her mouth. Most afternoons her eyes seem to blur and she feels a horrible rushing feeling washing over her head. When she gets home after leaving work early she finds she can't do much as she often feels dizzy, so tends to lie down.

Eight months ago Jane had a really bad episode and felt unwell on the bus and had to get off early. This happened a few times. She began to dread getting on the bus in case it happened again and so started walking to work. She didn't mind too much as she told herself it was good for her health to walk. Recently Jane was in a bar in town with friends when she had another similar experience and had to leave. She found this very embarrassing. Jane stopped going out in town with friends after this but still saw them locally. However, she has had to cancel arrangements with friends at the last minute because of her symptoms.

Jane is responsible for buying stock for the sandwich bar. She finds that for the last few weeks she can't face going to the supermarket for fear that she will collapse. She has asked someone else to do it instead. This is becoming a big problem for Jane, as it is her responsibility. Jane is becoming more worried and anxious about what is going on and realises that she has to do something.

The Five Areas assessment provides a clear summary of the range of difficulties you may face in each of the following areas:

- Physical symptoms/feelings in the body.
- Altered thinking (with extreme and unhelpful thinking).
- Altered feelings (also called moods or emotions).
- Altered behaviour or activity levels (with avoidance, reduced activity or unhelpful behaviours).
- Life situation, relationships, practical resources, problems and difficulties.

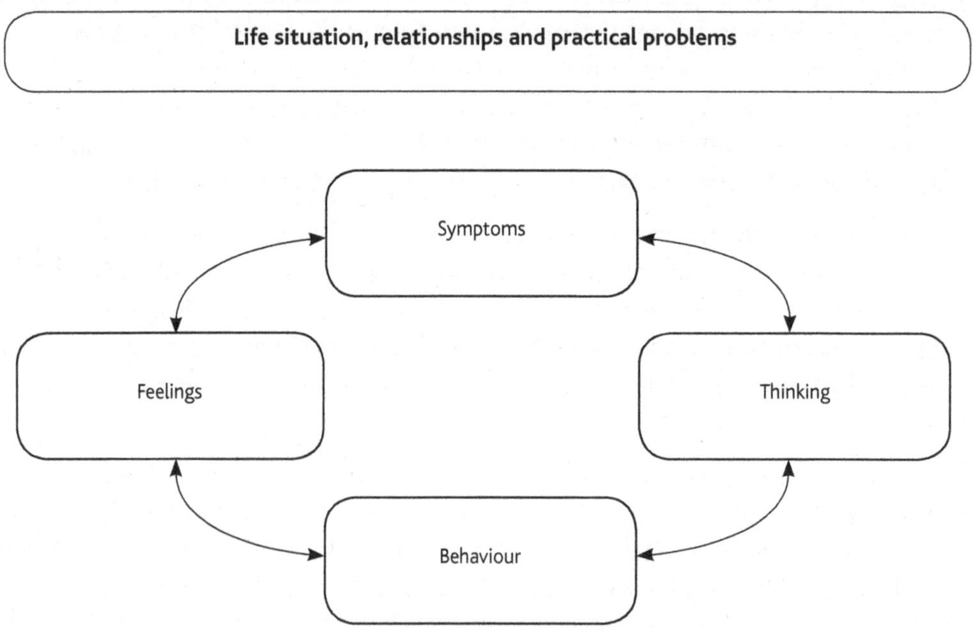

You have learned that what you think about a situation or problem may affect how you feel emotionally and physically. It also alters what you do. Because of the links between each of the areas, the actions that you take when you are worried or tense can act to worsen or keep your symptoms going.

The vicious circle of avoidance

Sometimes people avoid going into places and situations where they feel their symptoms might get worse. You may also stop doing certain things either because of symptoms or your worries about them. For example, people who feel uncomfortable in shops will avoid going into larger, busier ones. Similarly, someone who is worried about feeling dizzy will try to avoid any situations where they have felt dizzy before. So if you notice that your symptoms seem to get worse on a hot, crowded bus you might try to avoid going on buses.

This avoidance adds to your problems because although you may feel less anxious or unwell in the short term, in the longer term such actions worsen the problem. A **vicious circle of avoidance** may result. The problem with avoidance is that it teaches you the unhelpful rule that the only way of dealing with a difficult situation is through avoiding it. The avoidance also reduces the opportunities to find out that your worst fears do *not* occur. It therefore worsens anxiety and further undermines confidence. The process is summarised in the diagram below.

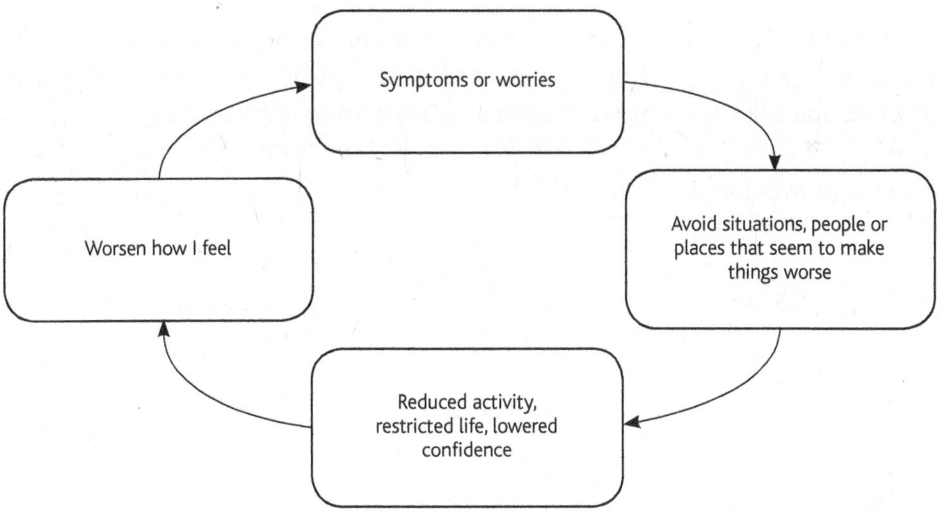

The vicious circle of avoidance.

To see if this applies to you, ask yourself 'What have I stopped doing because of how I feel?' Remember that at times the avoidance can be quite *subtle*: for example choosing to go to the shops at a time you know they are quiet, and then rushing through the shopping as quickly as possible, or just buying essentials.

What am I avoiding?

These questions will help you to think about the things you have stopped doing:

- Are there situations at work or in my relationships with others that I am avoiding?
- Is there anywhere I feel I can't go or anything I can't do because of my symptoms or worry about symptoms? Is this avoidance excessive or unnecessary?
- Do I avoid mixing with others? Is there anyone I am avoiding?
- Is this because of stress and worry or do I have other issues with them?
- What would I be able to do if I wasn't feeling like this? Am I avoiding things more subtly?

Write your answers to these questions here:

The checklist below will help you to think about your avoidance in greater detail. It summarises common areas that are avoided. If avoidance is a problem for you, it is likely that you will have noticed changes in at least some of these areas.

Checklist of avoidance

Am I:	
Avoiding walking alone away from home?	☐
Avoiding situations, objects, places or people because of fears about what harm might result?	☐
Avoiding physical activity or exercise because of concerns about my health?	☐
Avoiding dealing with important practical problems?	☐
Not really being honest with others, e.g. saying yes when I really mean no?	☐
Trying hard to avoid situations that bring about upsetting thoughts or memories?	☐
Brooding over things and no longer living life to the full?	☐
Avoiding opening or replying to letters or bills?	☐
Sleeping in to avoid doing things or meeting people?	☐

Avoiding answering the phone or the door?	☐
Avoiding sex?	☐
Avoiding being in crowded or hot places?	☐
Avoiding talking to others face to face?	☐
Avoiding going on buses, in cars, taxis, etc. or any place where it is difficult to escape?	☐
Avoiding busy or large shops?	☐
Other (write in)	

Sometimes the avoidance can be quite subtle and difficult to recognise. In fact you might even think that this behaviour is helpful to you. Now complete the following checklist..

Checklist: Unhelpful behaviours leading to subtle avoidance

Am I:	
Quickly leaving any situations?	☐
Rushing though a task as quickly as possible (e.g. walking or talking faster)?	☐
Trying very hard not to think about upsetting thoughts/memories? Trying to distract myself to improve how I feel?	☐
Only going out and doing things when others are there to help?	☐
Using medication differently to how it is prescribed to block how I feel or help me sleep, etc. (e.g. taking an extra dose)?	☐
Always carrying back-up medication 'just in case'?	☐
Taking the easiest option (for example joining the shortest queue in the shop or turning down opportunities that seem scary)?	☐
Deliberately looking away during conversations and avoiding eye contact? Bringing conversations to a close quickly because of not knowing what to say?	☐
Keeping so busy there is no time to stop, think and reflect on things?	☐
Avoiding things in other subtle ways? Write in other things you are doing, if this applies to you.	

Having completed these questions, reflect on your answers using the three questions below:

Q 1. Am I avoiding anything?

Yes ☐ No ☐

2. Has this reduced my confidence in things and led to an increasingly restricted life?

Yes ☐ No ☐

3. Overall, has this worsened how I feel?

Yes ☐ No ☐

Choice point

If you have answered 'Yes' to the above questions, then avoidance is likely to be a problem for you. You may like to focus on these areas and have a look at how to plan ways to overcome this.

Example: Kate recognises her avoidance

You have already met Kate in Workbook 2. Let's have another look at her situation.

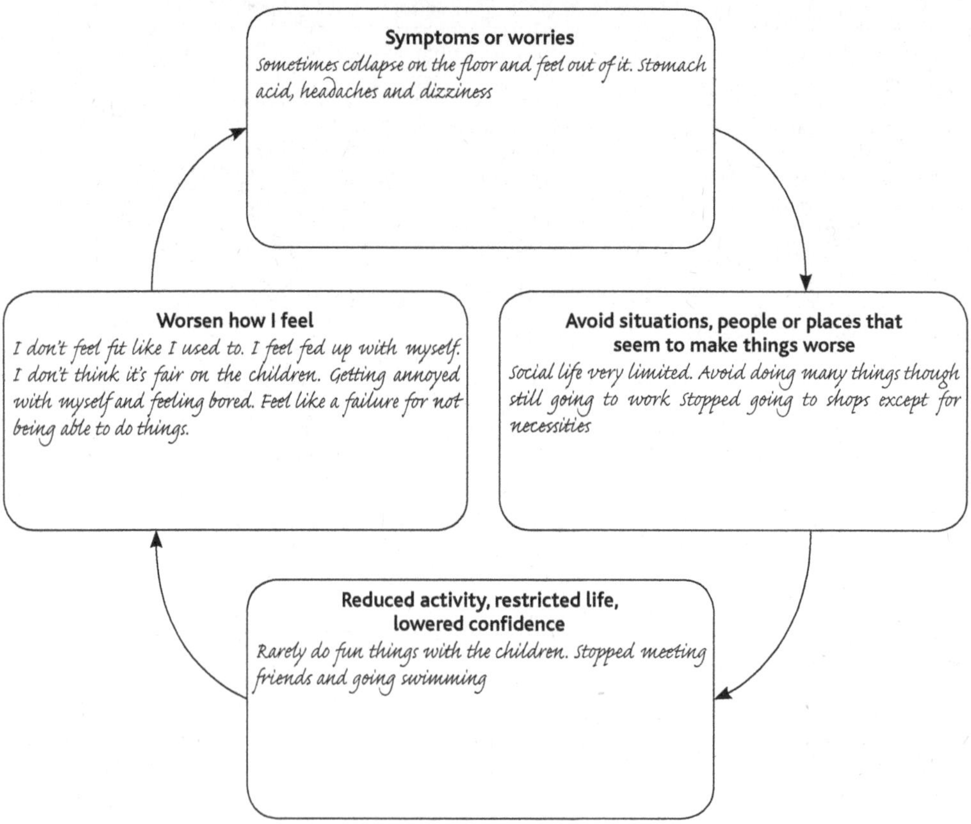

Kate's vicious circle of reduced activity and avoidance.

Kate is likely to feel better if she can break the vicious circle by:

- Slowly reintroducing things back into her life that give her a sense of pleasure and achievement. These must be activities that are realistic for her.
- Looking at ways of re-building the life she used to have by tackling her avoidance.
- An example of how she puts her plan into action can be found on page 129.

SECTION 4: Overcoming reduced activity

REMEMBER

If you haven't done this already, now is a good time to fill out an activity diary. You can find out how to do this in the Toolbox on pages 211 to 214.

David has completed a diary and gathered this background information. Now he can move on to use the **seven-step plan**. You will find out more about this as you go through this workbook. Exact instructions on how to make one for yourself are given in the Toolbox.

David's step-by-step approach

Step 1: Identify the activity to build on

David has already kept an **activity diary** for a week. The diary shows that the amount of pleasure David experiences varies during the day. What he does seems to affect how he feels. His activity diary helps him realise that he is happiest when he does things such as walking round the garden. He also had a sense of achievement with some other activities such as re-wiring a plug.

Example: David's activity diary for Tuesday morning

[6–7 am]	*[In bed asleep]*		(P)	(A)
7–8 am	*Woke up and listened to the radio*	*30 min*	2	2
8–9 am	*Got up and had a shower, cleaned my teeth*	*40 min*	*5*	*6*
9–10 am	***Made a coffee and breakfast***	*15 min*	*3*	*5*
10–11 am	*Re-wired a plug*	*45 min*	*6*	*7*
11–12 pm	*Watched television*	*50 min*	*3*	*5*
12–1 pm	*Walked round the garden*	*10 min*	*8*	*8*

The scale used by David to rate his enjoyment/pleasure (P) and achievement (A)

0	**5**	**10**
No pleasure/ achievement	Feel okay/ reasonable	Maximum pleasure/ achievement

Step 2: Choosing a target
It is important that David chooses a target problem that is likely to be helpful and achievable.

Example: David's target

David decides he should try to *increase the distance he walks*. He currently only ever walks as far as the car or round his small garden. He would like to be able to walk further.

Compare David's target – 'increase the distance I walk' – against the first three **questions for effective change**.

Questions for effective change

1. Will it be useful for understanding or changing how he is?

Yes ✓ No ☐

2. Is it a **specific task** so that he will know when he has done it?

Yes ☐ No ✓

3. Is it **realistic**: is it practical and achievable for him?

Yes ☐ No ✓

David's plan is helpful but it is *not specific* enough yet. It doesn't tell him *what* to do or define the steps needed to reach the goal. Planning this degree of detail is the next step for him to work on.

Step 3: Think up as many solutions as possible to plan this next step
David needs to look at the gap between what *he does now* and what he would like to do. He can bridge this gap by changing his activities in a number of really small steps. He should identify a clearly defined **first step** that he wants to do.

One difficulty that people often face is that they cannot see any way of changing things. A helpful way around this is to try to step back and come up with as many possible activities as possible. This approach is called **brainstorming**.

In brainstorming:

- The more solutions that are generated, the more likely it is that a good one will emerge.

- Ridiculous ideas should be included as well, even if you would never choose them in practice. This can help you to adopt a flexible approach to the problem.

So useful questions to help you to think up possible solutions are:

- What *ridiculous* solutions can I include as well as more sensible ones?
- What helpful ideas would others (e.g. family, friends or colleagues at work) suggest?
- What approaches have I tried in the past in similar circumstances?
- What advice would I give a friend who was trying to tackle the same problem?

Example: David's list of options

David sits with a piece of paper and thinks about possible ways he could start to increase the distance he walks. Read David's list below:

★ *Get Anne to drop me off miles away from the house and I'd have to walk home.*

★ *Walk around the golf course with my friend Jim.*

★ *Try to walk a bit further than I am just now.*

★ *Ask the doctor if a wheelchair or walking aid would be suitable.*

The aim here is to try and list as many potential activities as possible.

Step 4: Look at the advantages and disadvantages of each of the possible activities

The aim here is to examine the *pros* and *cons* of each potential activity that has been listed. Below is David's list of advantages and disadvantages for each activity he identified.

Suggestion	*Advantages*	*Disadvantages*
Get Anne to drop me off miles away from the house and I'd have to walk home	*I'd definitely be walking further than I am, it might just force me to do it*	*The idea is far too scary. I know I couldn't cope with it. Anyway Anne would never agree to it either*
Walk around the golf course with my friend Jim	*I like Jim and it would be nice to catch up. I love the golf course too*	*I'm not able to walk very far and it would be really embarrassing if I didn't manage it. Also it's an uneven surface which might not help*

Suggestion	Advantages	Disadvantages
Try to walk just a bit further than I am just now. Say 20 steps past the car	That doesn't sound too scary or too big a challenge	I'd be worried in case I let myself down or didn't manage it. Also I might collapse
Ask the doctor if a wheelchair or walking aid would be suitable	I'd be able to travel greater distances and meet up with friends at the shops	I'm definitely not that bad, I'm sure the doctor would have suggested it before if he thought it was a good idea. It might mean I was even less able to walk if I got too used to it

Step 5: Choose one of the solutions

The chosen solution should be realistic and likely to succeed. This decision will be based on your answers to step 3. David decides on option 3 – to try to walk just a bit further than he can now. Option 3 seems to be more realistic, practical and achievable. David reassures himself that if he did feel he might collapse he'd be close enough to home and any help that would be required.

KEY POINT

The solution that is chosen should be one that helps David tackle his target problem. It is important that he is realistic in his choice so that it does not seem impossible for him. You will see later how David can build upon this initial target for change with subsequent additional targets that will help him to progress.

Step 6: Plan the steps needed to carry it out

This is a key stage. Many people have some difficulty doing this to begin with. David needs to generate a clear plan that will help him to decide exactly *what* he is going to do and *when* he is going to do it.

It is useful for David to *write down* the steps needed to carry out the solution and to be specific about what he will do. This will help him to remember what to do and will allow him to predict possible problems that might arise. The questions for effective change should always be asked as part of this fifth step of the problem-solving approach, and can help David to re-check how practical and achievable his plan is.

Questions for effective change

Is the plan one that:

- Is **useful** for understanding or changing how I am?

- Is a **specific task** so that I will know when I have done it?
- Is **realistic**: is it practical and achievable?
- Makes clear *what* I am going to do and *when* I am going to do it?
- Is an activity that won't be easily blocked or prevented by practical problems?

The aim of these questions is to try to help David plan effectively what he is going to do.

Example: David reflects on the five questions for effective change:

1. Is it useful for understanding or changing how I am?

If I can manage to walk a further distance than I am at the moment it would change lots of things in my life.

2. Is it a specific task so that I will know when I have done it?

I'm clear what I am going to do – I'll start tomorrow morning.

3. Is it realistic: is it practical and achievable?

Is it realistic–yes, I can do that, I'd be lying if I didn't admit to myself that the idea scares me a bit because I don't know how I'll feel or how my legs will be, but it's really only a little bit scary – I am sure I can do this.

4. Does it make clear what I are going to do and when I am going to do it?

I'm starting at 11 am tomorrow morning. I already know I can walk as far as the car, so I'm going to try to walk 20 steps past the car onto the pavement in front of the house and back again.

5. Is it an activity that won't be easily blocked or prevented by practical problems?

Now then, what might block it? I guess if it's raining it might put me off but I'll just put on a jacket. If my legs feel really weak I can rest on the wall for a few minutes. The only other thing that I can predict could prevent me doing this is if I lose my nerve and try to put it off, but I think it will be alright and Anne knows what I'm going to try, so she'll be a support.

David's goals are now *clear and specific and his target is realistic*. He knows *what* he is going to do and *when* he is going to do it. He has predicted potential difficulties that might get in the way. This seems like a well thought through plan.

Step 7: Carry out the plan

Once David's plan is complete, he should act on it. On Tuesday morning David goes out and walks as far as the pavement. He feels uptight but manages this without major problem although his legs are shaky. He feels a real sense of achievement, as he has managed to walk further than he has for months.

Step 8: Review the outcome

David should look at what happened when he carried out his plan. How successful was the plan in tackling his original target problem 'to increase the distance I walk'?

Did his plan go smoothly, or were there any difficulties along the way? What has he learned from carrying out his plan?

David's review:

Q Was the selected approach successful?

Yes ✓ No ☐

Q Did it help me to increase the distance I walk (the target problem)?

Yes ✓ No ☐

Q Were there any disadvantages to using this approach?

Yes ☐ No ✓

What have I learned from what happened?

Example

That went really well. I know it wasn't very far but it was more than usual. Although my legs felt weak and shaky I still did it. I have learned that:

- *A specific written down plan can be helpful because I have talked about doing this before and not done it.*
- *My concerns about collapsing weren't true. I did feel uptight, but I noticed that when I did my last step I felt weak but pleased with my achievement.*

Building on what David has learned – putting together an activity plan

The next key stage is for David to build upon this first step so that he has a clear plan to move things forward. To do this, he needs to think about his *short-*, *medium-* and *longer-term targets*. The key is to build one step upon another, so that each time David plans out and completes the seven-step approach he can then consider what the next step will be. Without this sort of approach he may find that although he makes some progress, it's all in different directions and he will lose his focus and motivation. David summarises his activity plan below. Remember that each step can be planned out using the seven-step plan.

David also begins to *build in some other activities* to include tasks that also give him a sense of pleasure or achievement. For example doing some electrical work for Anne by changing a plug. The activities he chooses should be things that he values and sees as important.

Next steps: David's activity plan

Day and date	*Planned activity: Be specific. Is it a realistic plan? What do you have to do and when will you do it? What problems may occur? How can you overcome these problems?*	*Time*	*Pleasure (0–10) (P)*	*Sense of achievement (0–10) (A)*
Day 1, Tuesday, 11 am	Activity: Walk outside to the pavement, at least 20 steps but try a few more if possible.			
Day 2, Wednesday, 10 am	Rewire the other plug that Anne asked me to do weeks ago			
Day 2, Wednesday, 2 pm	After lunch walk at least 30 steps in the garden			
Repeat on Thursday				
Day 3, Friday, 11 am	Phone Jim and try to meet up with him next week			
Day 3, Friday, 2 pm	Walk to end of road, with Anne, have a rest and walk back			

The plan builds in at least several activities over the week that lead to a sense of pleasure. This can include both activities that build on his target area of increasing the distance he walks and also can include other activities as well.

Look back at the checklists on pages 109 to 110 and 118 to 119 to think of other things to include.

The key is to do everything at the right pace, so that change happens, but not so quickly that it seems too fast or too scary.

The example used shows how the technique might be applied to David's situation. However, it also can be applied to alter *any* problem. Next we'll look again at Kate, who has chosen to focus on getting back to her swimming.

Kate's plan

Kate has found it increasingly difficult to socialise as she used to. She has also found shopping particularly difficult and has stopped going swimming – something that she used to enjoy. Now she is spending more and more time at home on her own.

Kate goes through the same seven steps that David used. The target that she initially chooses is to '*go to the local swimming pool*'. She then thinks up as many solutions as possible about a sensible first step, and weighs up the advantages and disadvantages of each.

She identifies that the advantage of going swimming will be to increase confidence and boost her fitness. The disadvantage might be that she begins to feel dizzy or has a seizure. Kate realises that in the last two years she has become much more able to tell when a fit might happen. On balance she judges that this target is realistic and achievable for her.

She uses the **Questions for effective change** to help her plan what she is going to do in detail. She decides the exact date (Monday) and time (6 pm) when she will do this, as she knows children's swimming lessons are finished at this time and the pool shouldn't be too busy. Kate sets her target of swimming four breadths of the pool and staying no longer than 30 minutes. In the past she swam 60 lengths every time she went so she realises that she may see the four breadths as being 'hardly anything'. She decides to challenge this thought if it occurs by saying to herself: '*This is just a first step – I'll get there in the end – enjoy what you're doing now.*'

Kate also predicts the things that might go wrong – so she decides that if she experiences any symptoms she will sit on the poolside and use some of the relaxation techniques she knows just in case the symptoms are being made worse by feeling uptight about swimming again.

Kate's initial plan in action

On Monday evening at 6 pm Kate goes swimming. She admits to herself that she has spent the day worrying about what might go wrong but finally persuades herself to give it a go. Kate feels strange about being in the pool after such a long time away but enjoys her first swim. She finds that she tires very easily and sensibly changes her target of four breadths to three and manages to do this.

When she gets home, she reviews what she has done. Feeling very satisfied Kate then plans the next steps. These can be seen on Kate's **activity plan**.

Next steps: Kate's activity plan

Day and date	*Planned activity: Be specific. Is it a realistic plan? What do you have to do and when will you do it? What problems may occur? How can you overcome these problems?*	*Time (mins)*	*Pleasure (0–10) (P)*	*Sense of achievement (0–10) (A)*
Day 1, Monday, 6 pm	*Go to the swimming pool and swim four breadths. On review: she managed three breadths*			
Day 3, Wednesday, 6 pm	*Go to the swimming pool and again swim three breadths*			
Day 6, Saturday, 11 am	*Ask her daughter to come swimming. Don't need to set a target amount, just be comfortable in pool with company – but plan to stay no more than 35 minutes*			

SECTION 5: Overcoming avoidance

Earlier in this workbook we described Jane's situation: it was clear that she has several areas of avoided activity. Although in this example Jane has chosen to focus on her fear of shopping in supermarkets, the same principles can be applied to any avoided activities.

Checklist: Identifying Jane's avoidance

Am I:	**Tick here if you have noticed this**
Avoiding walking alone far from home?	
Avoiding situations, objects, places or people because of fears about what harm might result?	✓ *I get so dizzy and I can't focus. I might fall down. I may stop breathing during the panic*
Avoiding physical activity or exercise as a result of concerns about my physical health?	✗
Avoiding dealing with important practical problems (both large and small)?	✗
Not really being honest with others. For example, saying yes when I really mean no?	✗
Trying hard to avoid situations that bring about upsetting thoughts/memories?	✗
Brooding over things and therefore not longer living life to the full?	✗
Avoiding opening or replying to letters or bills?	✗
Sleeping in to avoid doing things or meeting people?	✗
Avoiding answering the phone, or the door when people visit?	✗
Avoiding sex?	✗
Avoiding talking to others face to face?	✗
Avoiding being with others in crowded or hot places?	✓ *I don't go out with my friends to bars any more*

Am I:	**Tick here if you have noticed this**
Avoiding busy or large shops, or finding that I have to think about where and when I go shopping, etc.?	✓ *I'm not going to large shops at all now. I definitely couldn't go to a supermarket because I'd get panicky. I'd feel really hot and sweaty and start breathing very fast. I'd be scared I'd collapse*
Avoiding going on buses, in cars, taxis, etc., or any places where it is difficult to escape?	✓ *I always walk to work now*

She also thinks about whether she is avoiding things in more subtle ways.

Examples of subtle avoidance

Unhelpful behaviours leading to subtle avoidance.

Am I:	
Quickly leaving any situations?	✓ *I have left one shop really quickly. I just left the trolley in the middle of the store and ran*
Rushing through a task as quickly as possible? (e.g. walking or talking faster)?	✓ *I definitely rush round the shop to get it over with as soon as possible*
Trying very hard not to think about upsetting thoughts/ memories. Trying to distract myself to improve how I feel?	✗
Only going out and doing things when others are there to help?	✗
Using medication differently to how it is prescribed to block how I feel or help me sleep etc. (e.g. taking an extra dose)?	✓ *Sometimes I take extra puffs of my inhaler*
Always carrying back-up medication 'just in case'?	✗

Am I:	
Taking the easiest option (e.g. joining the shortest queue in the shop or turning down opportunities that seem scary)?	✓ *I go to the small local shops at the quietest possible time. I always choose the shortest queue because of anxiety rather than because it is the obvious choice*
Deliberately looking away during conversations and avoiding eye contact. Bringing conversations to a close quickly because of not knowing what to say?	✗
Am I avoiding things in other subtle ways? Write in what you are doing here if this applies to you.	✓ *I grip hard onto the trolley when I feel anxious*

On answering the following three questions Jane determines that she is experiencing a **vicious circle of avoidance**.

Q 1. Am I avoiding doing things as a result of anxiety?

Yes ✓ No ☐

Q 2. Has this reduced my confidence in things and/or led to an increasingly restricted life?

Yes ✓ No ☐

Q 3. Overall, has this worsened how I feel?

Yes ✓ No ☐

Jane has very clear areas of avoidance (going into larger shops/supermarkets, buses and busy bars). She has also identified some more subtle problems of avoidance that need to be built into her plan.

Jane then uses the seven-step approach to overcome her avoidance.

Jane's seven-step approach

Step 1: Identify and clearly define the problem as precisely as possible

The important first step is identifying a *single* initial target area that she wants to focus on. This should be *clearly defined*. This step is particularly important as Jane has identified three main problems of avoidance (hot and crowded places, going to large shops/supermarkets and buses). It is not possible to overcome both these areas at once. Instead she needs to decide which *one* area to focus on to begin with. This means putting the other area on one side for the time being.

Jane writes down the specific area of avoided activity that she is going to focus on to start with.

Example: Jane's target area

Tackling my avoidance of large and busy shops/supermarkets.

Step 2: Think up as many solutions as possible to achieve this goal

The purpose of brainstorming is to try come up with as many ideas as possible. Among them Jane hopes to be able to identify a realistic, practical and achievable first step towards overcoming her problem.

Example: Jane's possible solutions

Jane sits and thinks about possible ways she could begin to start going into large and busy shops again:

- *Contact the manager of the supermarket and pay them a lot of money to arrange a personal evening opening when I can shop alone.*
- *Go into the largest, busiest shop I can find and stay there until I feel better.*
- *Take part in a sponsored shop for charity.*
- *Plan a slow increase in going to shops. Go to a local, smaller shop first. Begin to face my fears by slowing down my shopping and not racing round the store.*
- *Go to the post office at the busiest time and join the longest queue.*

Step 3: Look at the advantages and disadvantages of each of the possible solutions

Jane assesses how effective and practical each potential solution is. This involves considering the advantages and disadvantages for each potential solution.

Example: Jane thinks of the pros and cons

Suggestion	*Advantages*	*Disadvantages*
Contact the manager of the supermarket and pay them a lot of money to arrange a personal evening opening when I can shop alone	*I'd be able to go shopping without anyone else there. It would make me feel like a VIP*	*That's one of those ridiculous ideas you're supposed to think up in brainstorming. It would cost a fortune. I can't afford that sort of thing. Anyway, I'd feel like a right idiot asking for this. I'm not at all sure the shop would go along with this sort of arrangement*
Go into the largest, busiest shop I can find and stay there until I feel better	*That's a really unattractive option. I'm not sure it would work, and there don't seem to be many advantages I can think of!*	*Although I've heard that sort of approach can sometimes work, there is just no way I am going to do this. It is just too scary*
Take part in a sponsored shop for charity	*It would raise some money for charity*	*I just don't fancy this at all. Everyone would know what I was doing. I'd let people and the charities down if I couldn't do it. That would just make me feel like I'd failed. It's just too scary to do*
Plan a slow increase in going to shops. Go to a local, smaller shop first. Begin to face my fears by slowing down my shopping and not racing round the store	*This is something I can do without getting too panicky. It would be a really good first step. I could build up my confidence doing this first and then begin to go to larger, busier shops*	*The local shop doesn't stock all the food I like. It also costs a lot more than the supermarket. I don't want to have to keep shopping there. I want to be able to go to the supermarket*

Suggestion	Advantages	Disadvantages
	and the supermarket. It would boost my confidence. This could be the first small step in getting back to normal	
Go to the post office at the busiest time and join the longest queue	*I want to be able to do that. I post a lot of letters to friends*	*It might be a little too scary. I go there anyway, but the idea of going when it is really busy and then joining the longest queue is too much at the moment. It's just too ambitious*

Step 4: Choose one of the solutions

Jane's chosen solution should be an option that will address her problem. It should be realistic and likely to succeed. Jane's decision is based on the answers to step 3. Jane decides on option 4: '*Plan a slow increase in going to shops. Go to a local, smaller shop first. Begin to face my fears by slowing down my shopping and not racing round the store.*'

This solution is an option that fulfils the following two questions for effective change:

Q 1. Is it helpful?

Yes ✓ No ☐

Q 2. Is it realistic, practical and achievable?

Yes ✓ No ☐

Step 5: Plan the steps needed to carry it out and apply the questions for effective change

This is a key stage. Jane needs to generate a clear plan that will help her to decide exactly *what* she is going to do and *when* she is going to do it. It is useful for Jane to *write down* the steps needed to carry out the solution. This will help her to plan what to do and allows her to predict possible blocks and problems that might arise.

The **questions for effective change** can help Jane to re-check how practical and achievable her plan really is.

1. Will it be useful for understanding or changing how I am?

Example

I can go to small, local shops at the moment. I try to go at quieter times like the early afternoon, and then rush round. If I could change that rushing around, that would be an important first step.

2. Is it a specific task so that I will know when I have done it?

Example

I need to be clear about what I am going to do. I will go shopping as I normally do. Instead of just shooting round the shop and grabbing the things I need, I will try to walk round it at a slower pace. I'll know I've done this if I look at my watch just before I go into the shop, and again just after I leave. I want to stay in there at least 10 minutes to begin with.

3. Is it realistic; is it practical and achievable?

Example

Is it realistic? Yes, I can do that. It's really only a little bit scary. I'm sure I can do this.

4. Does it make clear what you are going to do and when you are going to do it?

Example

I have a clear idea of what I need to do. I will spend at least 10 minutes in the shop. I need to think about how I can spend the extra time there. I could look for some other provisions, or read the ingredient labels. Even better, I could stop at the DVD stand and look at what films they have in. That's something that could take a few minutes. I need to decide when I am going to do this trip to the shops. I think I should do it on Tuesday at 2pm.

5. Is it an activity that won't be easily blocked or prevented by practical problems?

Example

Now then, what might block it? If the shop was very busy, I might want to leave more quickly. I could plan to go at a quieter time of day, and even if there are a few people there, I could choose to stay. The only other thing that I can predict could prevent me doing this is if I lose my nerve and try to start rushing round when I get there. If I have that temptation, I just need to make sure I slow down my breathing, and also my walking. I'll deliberately not leave the shop, and just stay there for a few more minutes before leaving. I know from before that I'm going to notice my usual fear that 'I will collapse'. I need to be aware of that and try to challenge these fears.

Jane's goals are *clear, specific and her target is realistic*. She knows *what* she is going to do and *when* she is going to do it. She has predicted potential problems that might get in the way. This seems like a well thought through plan.

Step 6: Carry out the plan

Jane carries out her plan

Jane goes to the shop the next day. Before she enters the shop, she notes her anxious thoughts down on a piece of paper and records how much she believes them. She reminds herself that as she carries out the plan this will help undermine the old fears.

Before she goes into the shop, she notices the fear that *I will collapse*. She believes this 30 per cent at the time. She records her anxiety as being 30 per cent as well. She challenges it by reminding herself that she never has collapsed.

When she goes into the shop, there are three other people already there. They are an older couple and a school child. Her belief that she will collapse shoots up to 80 per cent. She rates herself as 70 per cent anxious. She thinks about leaving and begins to feel a pressure in her chest and hot and sweaty. She notices an increase in both her heart rate and breathing and starts to feel dizzy – her eyesight also begins to blur. She begins to walk faster to try to get all her shopping done as quickly as possible. She then remembers that she had decided that if she felt like this she would try to control her breathing and slow down her walking.

Jane makes a big effort and stops in the aisle by the magazines. She picks one up and flicks through it. She does this for a couple of minutes, and begins to feel much better. Her anxiety and belief that she will collapse both slowly drop to around 40 per cent. She is able to complete the rest of her shopping at a normal pace. When she leaves the shop, she is surprised to find that she has been in there for almost 20 minutes.

Step 7: Review the outcome

Jane should next review what happened when she carried out her plan. Did it go smoothly, or were there any difficulties along the way? What has she learned from carrying out the plan?

Jane's review

Was the selected approach successful?

Yes ✓ *No* ☐

Did it help start to overcome the problems of avoidance during shopping (the target problem)?

Yes ✓ *No* ☐

Were there any disadvantages to using this approach?

Yes ☐ No ✓

What have I learned from what happened?

That went really well. I was almost thrown though when there were three people already in the shop. That hardly ever happens.

The three things I have learned are:

1. Just how useful it is to have predicted what to do if I began to feel worse. When that happened I felt really scared. I remembered that I had planned to slow down my breathing and my walking if that happened. It worked! I felt a lot better – especially after looking at the DVDs.

2. All my concerns about collapsing if I stayed in just weren't true. I did feel anxious when I went in – especially when I noticed the others there. However, the anxiety quickly began to fall as time passed. It didn't just keep going up and up like I thought it would.

3. Although at the time when I felt most anxious, I believed the fears that 'I'm going to collapse', the fear and physical sensations did not continue rising. I didn't collapse and when I think back – I never have collapsed while shopping.

KEY QUESTION

What does this say about any fears before or during the activity?

Jane reviews what happened to her fears and level of anxiety as she went round the shop.

Example

Well I didn't collapse. The fears just weren't right. I did feel bad at one stage, but I stuck with it and nothing bad happened. Amazing! I certainly believe that I'll collapse far less than before.

Task

Jane wrote down her extreme and unhelpful thoughts and recorded how much she believed them (from 0 – not at all, to 100 – believing them fully).

My fearful thought: '*I will collapse.*'

I believed this:

- 30 per cent *before* going into the shop.
- 80 per cent *during* the time in the shop when she saw all those people there. It then slowly dropped to 40 per cent.
- 10 per cent five minutes *after* leaving the shop.

Jane also records her level of anxiety at the time (from 0 – no anxiety, to 100 maximum anxiety).

Jane's level of anxiety:

- 30 per cent *before* going into the shop.
- 70 per cent *during* the time in the shop when she saw all those people there. It then slowly dropped to 40 per cent.
- 15 per cent five minutes *after* leaving the shop.

KEY POINT

Be aware of any extreme and unhelpful thinking both *before*, *during* and *after* your own planned task. These thoughts can cause stress and worry. The best way to undermine an extreme and unhelpful thought is to act against it.

In spite of the high levels of anxiety, Jane succeeded in her plan. She also noticed something else that is very important. Even though she felt 70 per cent anxious just after entering the shop, after only a few minutes the level of anxiety quickly began to fall. Her fear that she would collapse also dropped to only 40 per cent. By the time she left the shop and reflected on what happened, her belief in the original fearful thought had dropped to only 10 per cent. Facing up to fearful thoughts is a very good way of testing and challenging them.

By repeating the same activity *again and again* over the next week, Jane's fear becomes less and less intense. It also lasts for shorter and shorter lengths of time. By repeatedly facing her fears she is able to challenge her thoughts and reduce her anxiety. You can read more about this in Workbook 5.

Facing up to fear causes it to slowly lose its impact. This is illustrated in the diagrams below.

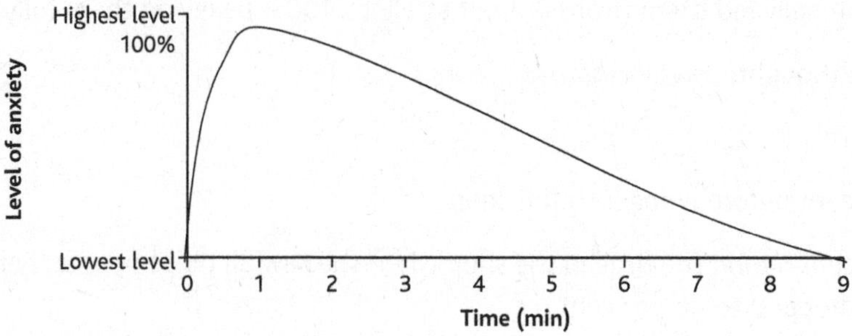

First time Jane faces her fears: Tuesday at 2 pm.

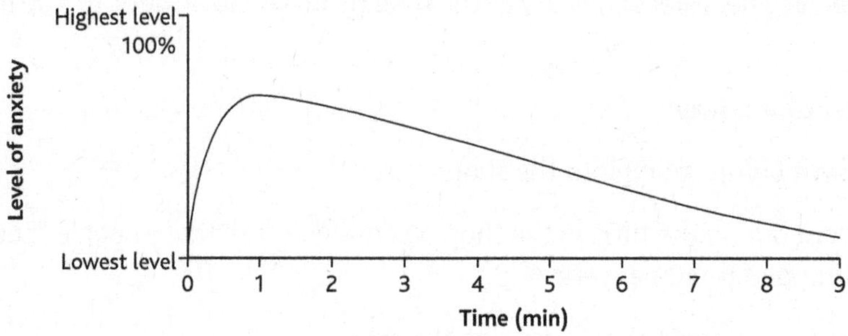

Second time Jane faces her fears: Wednesday at 11.30 am.

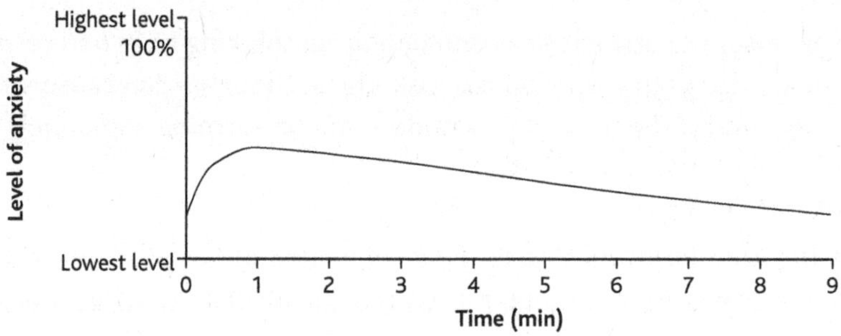

Third time Jane faces her fears: Friday at 3 pm.

SECTION 6: Building on the initial change using a step-by-step approach

The next stage is for Jane to build upon her initial step so that she has a clear plan to move things forward to the next step. To do this, she needs to think about her *short-, medium- and longer-term* targets/goals. The key is to build one step upon another, so that each time Jane plans out and completes the seven-step approach, she can consider what next step she will take. Each step should move her closer towards her target. Without this step-by-step approach she might lose her focus and motivation.

Jane plans out the different steps that she needs to complete over the next few weeks. Her plan should also include reducing and stopping doing any of the more subtle types of avoidance she has noticed.

Example

Jane's step-by-step weekly targets	*Initial fear level (0–100 per cent)*	*Time scale*
1. Going into the local shop for a paper. Walking round slowly, and staying there for at least 10 minutes	*Hardly scary at all 5–10 per cent scary*	*Week 1 and then repeat at least twice that week*
2. Going into the local shop. Deliberately choosing a busier time of day, and again to walk round slowly, staying in the shop for at least 20 minutes each time	*A little scary 15 per cent scary*	*Week 2 Repeat at least twice that week*
3. Queuing in the post office and deliberately choosing the longest queue	*Quite scary 35 per cent scary*	*Week 3 and then repeat at least twice that week*
4. Going into the supermarket foyer area to buy a newspaper and staying there for at least 20 minutes	*Pretty scary 50 per cent scary*	*Week 4 and 5 and then repeat at least twice each week*
5. Going into the supermarket at a quieter time and shopping for at least 20 minutes. Relaxing my grip on the trolley	*Moderately scary 75 per cent scary*	*Week 6 and then repeat at least twice that week*

Jane's step-by-step weekly targets	*Initial fear level (0–100 per cent)*	*Time scale*
6. Going shopping in the supermarket at a busier time by myself for at least 20 minutes. Having a relaxed grip on the trolley all the time	*Very scary 85 per cent scary*	*Week 7 and then repeat at least twice that week*
7. Eventual target: going shopping in the supermarket at a busier time and deliberately choosing the longest checkout queue by myself. Spend at least 20 minutes in the shop	*Very very scary 100 per cent scary at first*	*Week 8 and then repeat at least twice that week*

You can see that Jane's plan is clearly made up of separate targets. Each new target builds upon the previous one to help Jane move forwards. At each stage she is able to further test out and disprove her original fear and worrying thought that she will collapse.

Over a number of weeks this can add up to a very significant total change in what she is able to do. In completing each step Jane needs to be careful that she doesn't subtly avoid facing up to her fear when she is in the shop. For example, she may be tempted to rush around the shop as quickly as possible, try to distract herself from her fears while in the shop, or only go shopping when accompanied by a friend so that she feels safer. Instead, she should walk round each shop deliberately slowly. She should plan to also relax her grip on the trolley. Each time she repeats the same step her anxiety will be less intense. It will also last for a shorter time than the time before.

Each step should be realistic, practical and achievable. By succeeding in these planned steady steps, real progress can be achieved. You will have a chance to practise this same seven-step plan yourself using the example in the Toolkit on page 200.

Jane's five common 'subtle' avoidances and five possible solutions

When shopping, deliberately go only when the shop is likely to be empty	Slowly plan to go to the shop at busier times. Eventually to go to busier and larger shops
Rushing round the shop as quickly as possible	Slow down the walking round the shop. Plan to deliberately stand and look at some of the goods. At a later stage deliberately choose to talk to an employee about a product

Choosing the smallest queue at the tills. The motivation here is to leave the shop as quickly as possible because of anxiety rather than just to be efficient	Choose to use longer queues and use methods of payment that take longer (e.g. paying by credit card)
Using *distraction techniques* to avoid noticing the anxiety when in the shop. For example, by doing *mental* arithmetic while in the shop, or completing a *physical* activity (such as clenching her fists tightly)	Choose to stop doing the distraction technique and pay attention to the task she is doing
Seeking reassurance and support from others when out shopping	Create a reassurance-free zone by beginning to do things with less and less reassurance from others

Anxiety and over-worry about health problems

You read about Naz in Workbook 2 – he has had problems with avoidance and anxiety since his symptoms started.

Example: Naz's problem of avoidance

After a collapse, Naz becomes convinced that he is likely to have a stroke. As a result he constantly feels anxious and is preoccupied with his illness. He feels physically tense and cannot sleep. He has stopped any activities that he fears may bring on a stroke such as doing exercise, and being at work.

This has led to concern and phone calls from work colleagues and pressure from his sister to do more to help their parents and has further added to his problems. His doctor has advised him that he needs to do some exercise in order to stay fit.

Naz's first step

- Eventual target to be achieved.

'*I want to be able to play five-a-side-football like I used to do.*'

- Main fear to be challenged.

'*I will have a stroke if I overdo things.*'

- Subtle avoidance to take into account in the plan.

'*I look in the mirror to see if I look pale. I only go places when someone else is around, whenever I notice my symptoms I check my blood pressure.*'

Naz's step-by-step weekly targets to increase the level of physical exercise	Time scale
1. Start out with brisk walk around the local area. Over the week repeat twice and increase the distance slowly. Continue to walk at a brisk pace. By the end of the week aim to be able to walk to the local shops. To start reducing my blood pressure monitoring to twice per day	Week 1 Repeat the walk on two more occasions this week
2. Go out for gentle jog, aim to run one minute, walk one minute and maintain this for 15 minutes, slowly build up. Reduce my blood pressure measuring to once per day	Week 2
3. Continue with jogging but try to increase intervals to a three-minute run and two-minute walk for 20-30 minutes	Week 3
4. Go along to five-a-side-football and play for just 10 minutes out of the hour but make a point of chatting to colleagues too. Stop monitoring blood pressure altogether. Just save it for when my doctor recommends a review.	Week 4 and 5
6. Eventual target: play five-a-side-football for at least 30 minutes and build this up over the coming weeks.	Week 6

Worries about your health are very natural but every now and again may get out of hand. As you have seen, sometimes your thoughts and behaviours only add to your original fears.

These worries can be tackled in the same way as all your other thoughts. You will find a way to do this in Workbook 5.

There are also a number of very common things that people start doing when they have symptoms. These are not helpful in the long term but may make you feel better in the short term.

- Scanning your body for any signs of illness can continue to reinforce fears about ill health.
- Sometimes walking in ways that are designed to protect against pain and stiffness actually worsens this by creating additional stresses on your body. Holding your muscles stiffly can lead to pulled muscles or cramps.
- Only going out with someone else 'just in case' you become ill. This teaches you the unhelpful rule that you can only cope with additional support.
- Taking a mobile phone because of anxious fears that you may need to call for help if you become ill.

- Using inhalers or tablets such as an anti-angina tablet or painkillers in a way they were not prescribed. For example, taking them before exercise even though this was not suggested or recommended to you.
- Walking slower or exercising less than usual as a result of health fears.
- Measuring your pulse to check it is strong and regular. Other ways of checking how you are can include looking in the mirror, feeling for lumps, etc.
- Doing daily health checks such as your blood pressure, temperature and pulse rate.
- Going to the doctor over aches or pains that have been investigated fully before.
- Asking for reassurance from others about how you look.
- Spending time either paying special attention to news items or information about health, or trying to avoid it altogether. Your aim should be a healthy balance here.
- Selectively listening to what other people say and picking out any small thing that might just relate to your health.
- Expecting others to do things for you that you are capable of doing yourself.
- Walking with a stick or using a wheelchair can sometimes add to difficulties. If possible, plan to reduce such aids unless advised otherwise by your healthcare practitioner. Specialist advice is sensible here.

You can use the same plans that you find in the Toolbox to slowly reduce these. Learn from Jane's approach of having short-, medium- and longer-term goals, and try to do this in a paced way.

My current goal

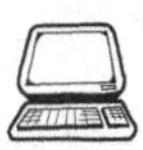

You can get additional help and support in problem solving at www.livinglifetothefull.com

Acknowledgements

The use of the Five Areas assessment model and associated language is used from the Overcoming Five Areas series by permission of Hodder Arnold Publishers and Dr C Williams. Illustrations are by Keith Chan and are reproduced with permission.

My notes

Workbook 5

Noticing and changing unhelpful thinking

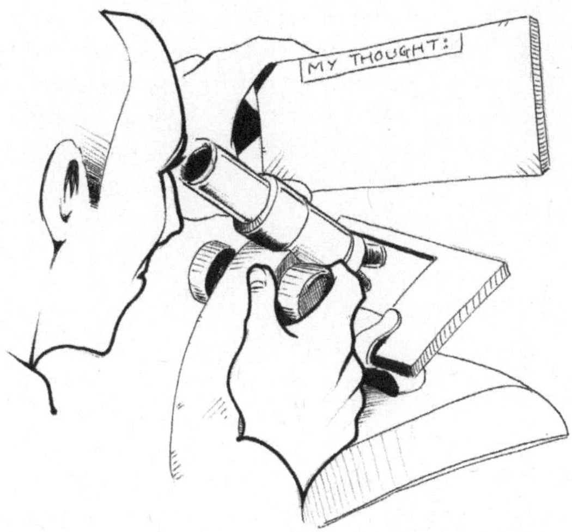

overcoming
functional neurological symptoms:
A Five Areas Approach

SECTION 1: Introduction

Symptoms can bring with them many frustrations, doubts and fears. If symptoms go on for some time you may begin to feel ground down by them. As a result your thinking can change. For example, you may start to experience unhelpful thoughts about:

- Your symptoms.
- Your current situation.
- Your future outlook.
- Those around you, including your family and friends, and your healthcare practitioners.

If your symptoms have continued in spite of medical consultations, it is not uncommon to feel frustrated, angry with, or misunderstood by doctors. You may also feel that your family and friends offer you less support than they did at first. To find out more about your responses to other people and their reactions towards you, see Workbook 3 and Toolbox E.

In this workbook you will learn about:

- **Noticing your thinking.**
- **Considering the unhelpful effect of some of these thoughts.**
- **How to question and change these thoughts.**
- **How to put what you've learned into practice.**

KEY POINT

You are more prone to unhelpful thinking when you feel sore, tired or upset.

Unhelpful thinking styles

The first step in changing unhelpful thinking is to start noticing how common it is in your own life. Often when you feel an emotion, it is linked to an unhelpful thought. However, being aware of your thinking doesn't mean that:

- You think like this all the time.
- You have to notice all of the unhelpful thinking styles.

Checklist of unhelpful thinking styles

Unhelpful thinking style	*Some typical thoughts*	*Tick if you have noticed this thinking style recently*
Putting a negative slant on things (negative mental filter)	I see things through dark-tinted glasses	☐
	I see the glass as being half empty rather than half full	☐
	Whatever I've done in the week it's never enough to give me a sense of achievement	☐
	I tend to focus on the bad side of everyday situations	☐
Jump to the worst conclusion (catastrophising)	I tend to predict that the very worst outcome will happen	☐
	I'm going to collapse	☐
	I'm going to end up in a wheelchair or worse	☐
Having a gloomy view of the future (make negative predictions)	I tend to predict that things will go wrong	☐
	If one thing goes wrong I often predict that everything will go wrong	☐
	I'm always looking for the next thing to fail	☐
	This is all hopeless, there's no point	☐
Putting myself down (bias against myself)	I'm very self-critical	☐
	I overlook my strengths	☐
	I see myself as not coping	☐
	I don't recognise my achievements	☐
	Other people would cope better than me with this	☐
Negative view about how others see me (mind-reading)	I mind-read what others think of me	☐
	I often think that others don't like me/think badly of me without evidence	☐
Bearing all responsibility	I think I should take the blame if things go wrong	☐
	I've brought this on myself. It's all my fault	☐
	I think I'm responsible for everyone else	☐
Making extreme statements/rules	I use the words 'always' and 'never' a lot to summarise things	☐
	If one bad thing happens to me I often say 'Just typical' because it seems this always happens	☐
	I make myself a lot of 'must', 'should', 'ought' or 'got to' rules	☐
	I should just be able to put all this behind me and return to normal	☐

> **KEY POINT**
> **Often you believe these thoughts just because they 'feel' true and because of how you're feeling. You may forget to check out how true these thoughts actually are.**

Why can extreme thinking be unhelpful?

Surveys show that everyone thinks like this sometimes. Usually you are able to ignore it but there are times when you can't. This can particularly affect you when you are unwell, making you notice and dwell on the thoughts more.

What you think can be very powerful – it affects how you feel and what you do. There are three important impacts of your thoughts, as shown below.

Unhelpful thinking causes →

Changes in symptoms
Symptoms can get worse

Unhelpful feelings
You may feel more down, guilty, upset, anxious, ashamed, stressed or angry

Unhelpful behaviour changes
You may stop or reduce what you normally do or start to avoid things that worry you or cause stress. On the other hand, you may start to act in ways that seem to help but which end up backfiring and worsen how you feel in the longer term

> **KEY POINT**
> **These unhelpful thinking styles show the main ways that thinking can become extreme and unhelpful. Extreme thinking is unhelpful because it can worsen how you feel emotionally, alter your symptoms and unhelpfully alter what you do.**

Images

People often think in pictures or images. Images are a form of thought and may be 'still' images (like a photograph), or are moving (like a video). Images may be in black and white or may be in colour. They may include:

- Predictions of bad things happening in the future: for example being totally disabled or even dying.

- Memories of past events, for example images of a situation which didn't go well.
- Thoughts about how your body is working (for example images of what you think may be happening to your hearts, lungs, muscles or liver).
- Images about how others will react, for example mind-reading that others don't understand or really believe you and having a picture in your head of their faces.

In summary, images can also show any of the unhelpful thinking styles.

The next step is to practise ways of noticing extreme and unhelpful thinking. To do this, you will need to act like a thought detective by carrying out a **thought investigation** of the times when your feelings or symptoms alter.

SECTION 2: Completing a thought investigation

HINT

In order to identify extreme or unhelpful thinking, try to watch for times when you *suddenly* feel worse (e.g. some symptoms feel worse, you feel sadder, or more anxious, upset or angry). Then ask 'What went through my mind then'.

Act like a detective

The questions on the following pages will help you begin to work out how extreme thinking may affect how you feel and what you do. Try to **act like a detective** to piece together bit by bit the factors that led up to you feeling worse.

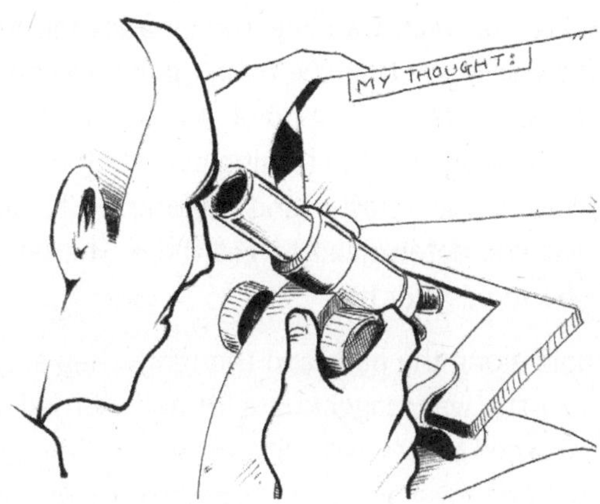

For this you first need to *think yourself back into the situation* when you felt worse. Try to slow down as you think back through the situation so that you can be as accurate as possible in your thought investigation. Second, try to **stop, think and reflect** as you consider the five different areas that can be affected. Now read this example of Caroline examining a time when she felt worse.

Example: Caroline's thought investigation of a time she had felt worse

Caroline has had symptoms for four years and over this time she has found ways to help her live with most of these. She tries very hard not to let symptoms interfere with her life. People are amazed by how much she does. At certain times, however, Caroline finds herself feeling really frustrated when things go wrong. Here is an example of one of those times.

It was a lovely spring Tuesday morning and Caroline had woken up feeling that she was going to have a good day. Once the children had gone to school she decided to take the dog for a walk. She tried to do this most days at around 10 am unless she woke up thinking it was going to be a bad day. She usually went to the local park and walked the same route.

To begin with she enjoyed being out in the sunshine and felt happy. As she walked she began to notice an ache in her leg around the knee. A few minutes later her leg felt heavy and started to get weak. Caroline immediately felt frustrated as she had been feeling good. She was angry that she wasn't going to complete her walk. She decided to push on to her usual turning point. As she walked she began to speed up and said to herself, 'I must get to the turning point before my leg gives out.' Her breathing and heart rate became faster and she started feeling dizzy and began to stagger but she was still determined to get there. She felt angry with herself because this used to be so easy for her.

Caroline noticed people along the path and thought, 'They are staring at me.' She was aware that by now she was staggering a lot and worried that 'they think I'm drunk'. She was also worried that 'I will fall over'. When Caroline finally got to the tree she was exhausted and miserable. Her symptoms slowly wore off but she had to sit down on the ground for some time before she could face the homeward journey. When she got home she cancelled her plans for the afternoon and felt disheartened.

When you first look at Caroline's day it is difficult to imagine what she could have done differently. She seems to be trying very hard and following advice to keep up with her normal activities as best she can. Now you are going to look at her story in more detail using the Five Areas Approach to see if Caroline could make any helpful changes.

The following steps help Caroline investigate for herself the five areas that may be linked to her upset. It helps to look in detail at:

- The situation, relationship or practical problems that occurred.
- Symptoms.
- Altered thinking (such as extreme or unhelpful thinking styles).
- Altered behaviour (such as reduced activity or starting to do unhelpful behaviours) that occurred.
- Altered feelings (also called moods or emotions).

You can look at these five areas in any order. Let's start with:

Area 1: Situation, relationship and practical problems (that is, the people and events around you)

Caroline writes a brief summary of the time/place, the people and the events happening when she begins to feel worse

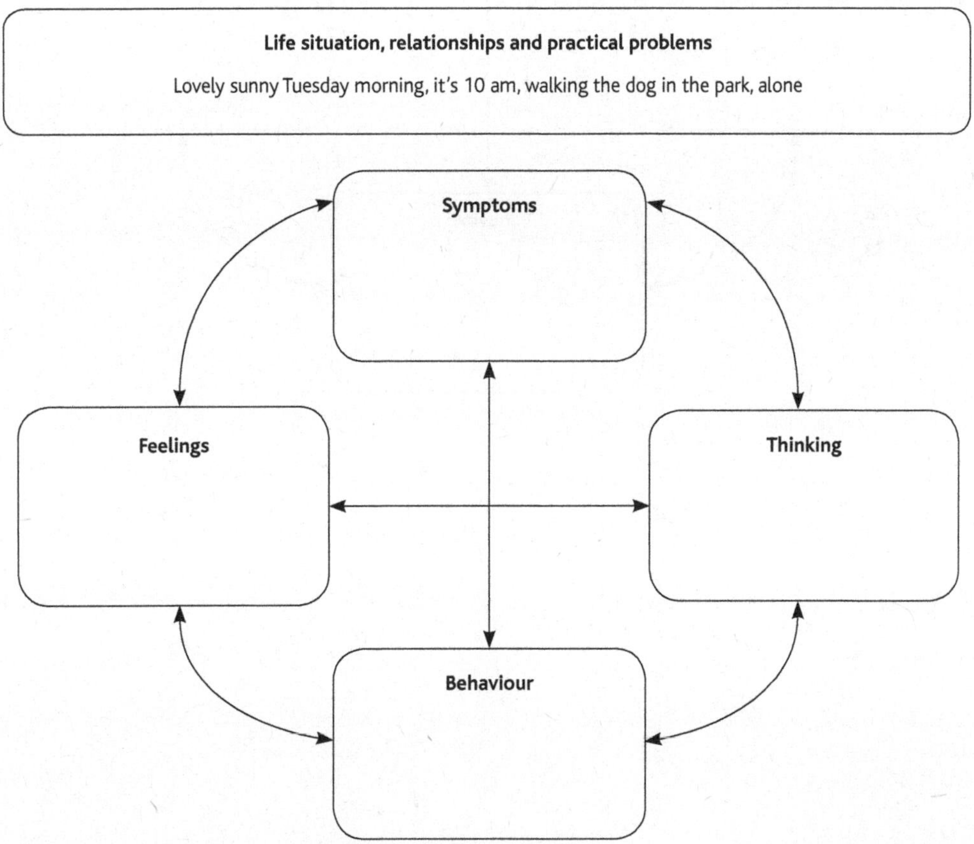

Area 2: Symptoms

Next let's look at how Caroline felt physically and fill this in on her Five Areas diagram.

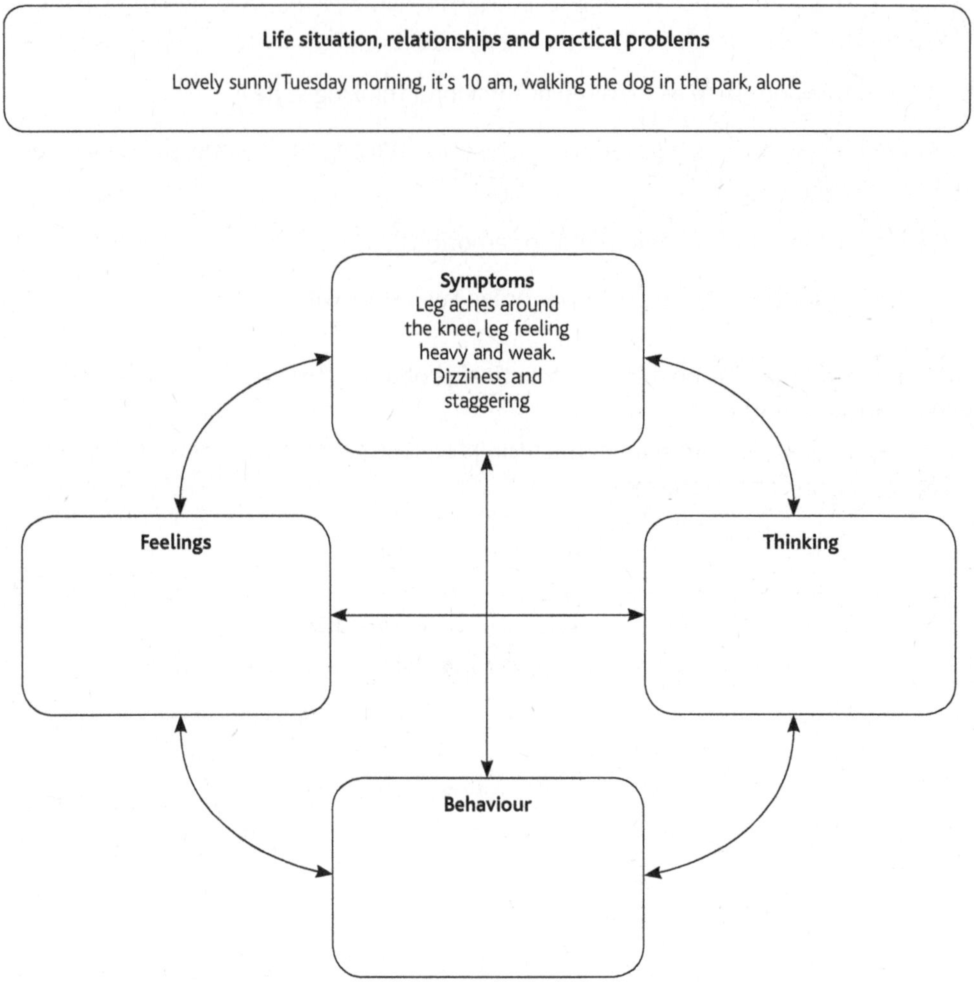

Area 3: Altered thinking

People are all different when it comes to how aware they are of their thoughts when they feel worse. This may be because the symptoms often overwhelm people's thoughts. In Caroline's case it was only later, when talking to her husband, that she realised that her frustration was made worse by the thought 'I *must* get to the turning point' and the thought 'or I will have failed' (an example of **making extreme statements/rules**). Caroline feared that people in the park would 'think I'm drunk' – an example of **mind-reading**. Caroline's husband asked her why she had pushed on but she couldn't really explain to him other than she thought she *must* reach the turning point or else she would have failed in some way (**bias against herself**).

Let's add these thoughts to Caroline's Five Areas diagram.

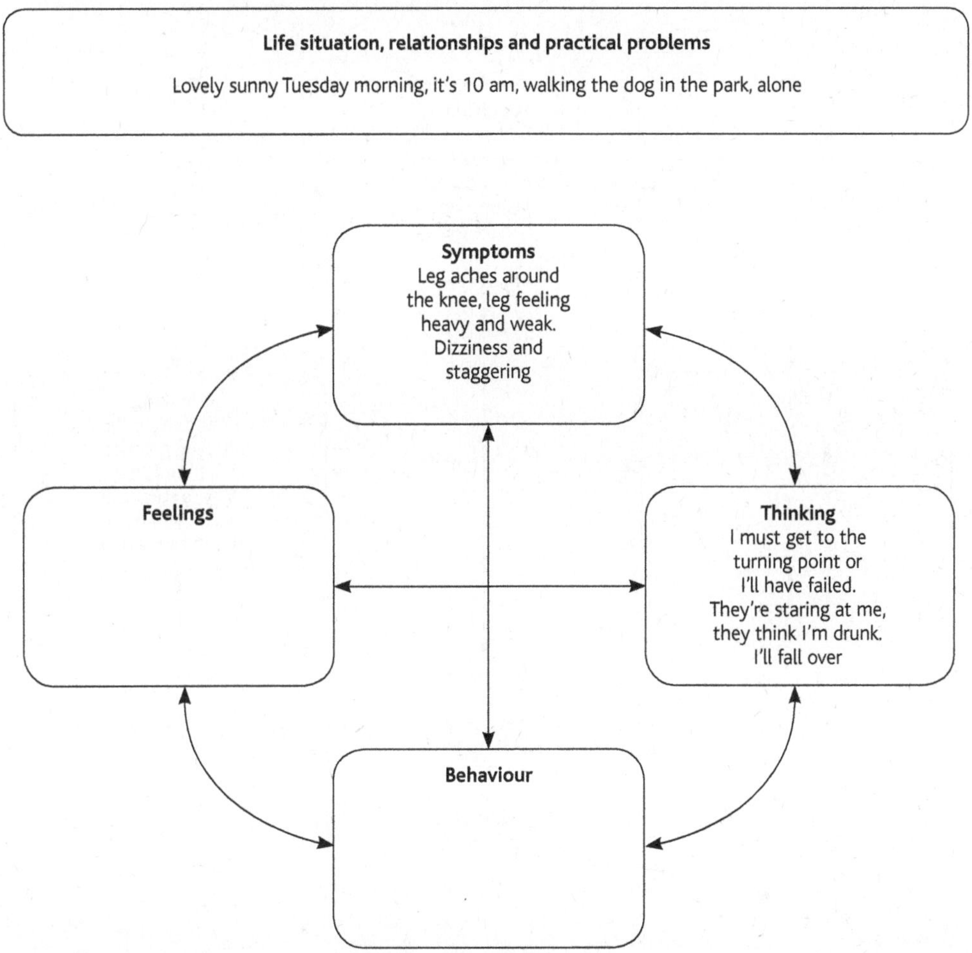

Area 4: Behaviour

Reading this example you can see how Caroline's symptoms and thoughts altered how she reacted. When she first noticed the symptoms she set herself a target that she *must* get to the turning point. She speeded up her walking pace and at the same time began to feel more and more upset as she began to struggle to get there. She ignored her worsening symptoms and fixed all her attention on getting to her target. Let's also add these in to her Five Areas diagram.

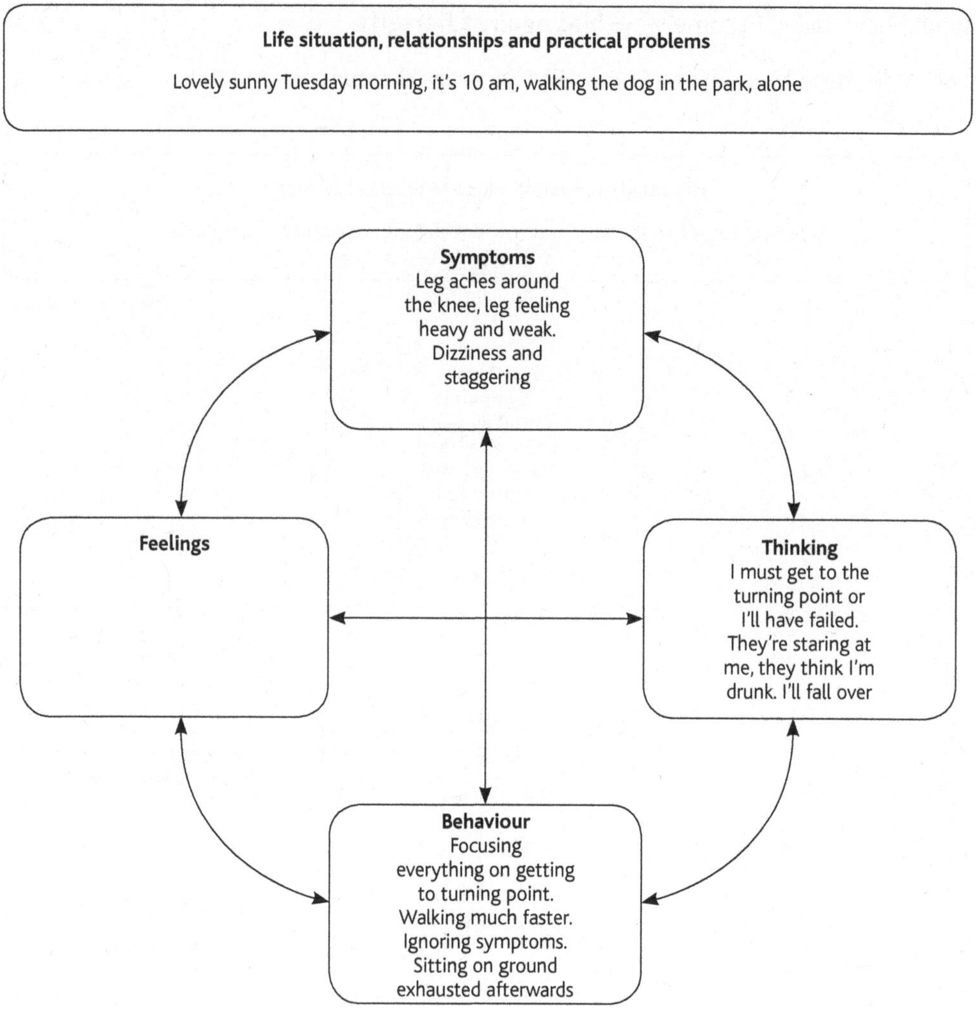

Area 5: Altered feelings emotions

Caroline had a number of feelings during her morning. She had initially really enjoyed her walk and it was a lovely sunny day. Once her symptoms began she felt increasingly frustrated and angry. She was worried about others' opinions of her. By the end she felt quite miserable and disheartened. You can now fill in your final box.

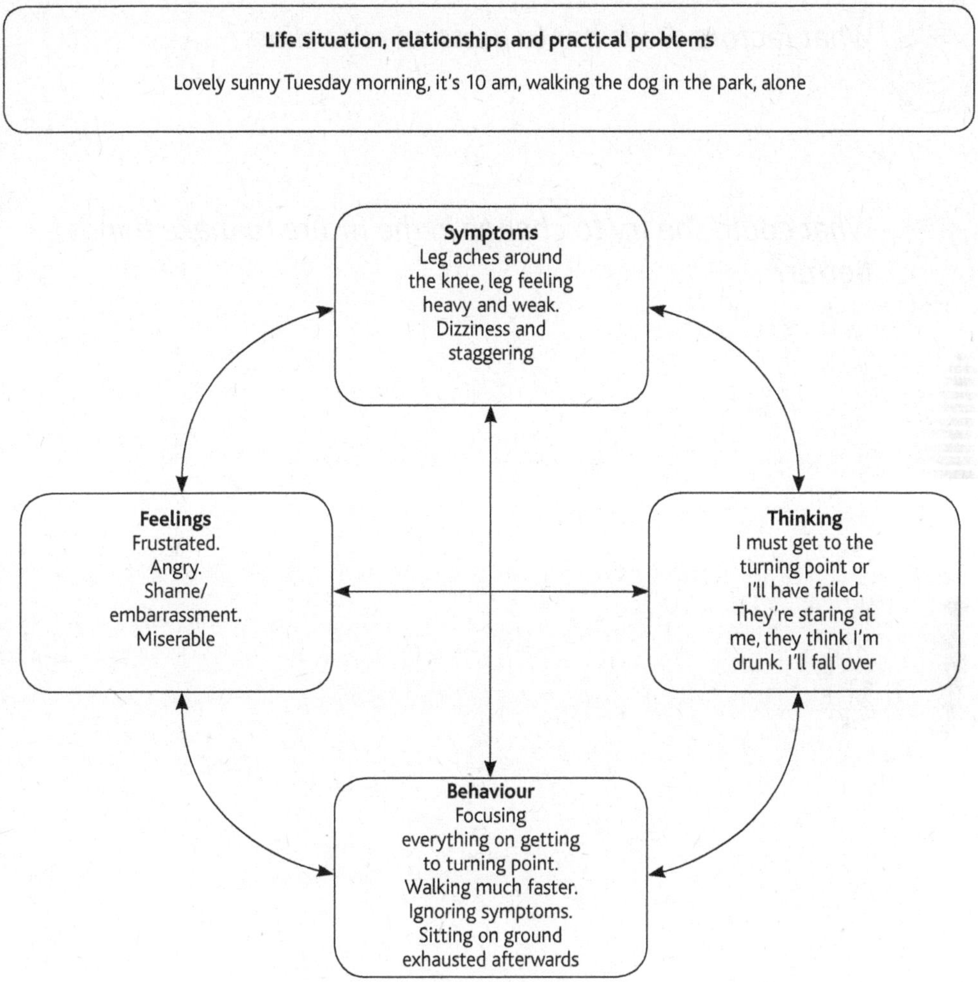

Caroline reflects on her thoughts. The thought that upset her most is: *I must get to the turning point or I'll have failed*. This thought is the **key thought** as it is the key to understanding why Caroline felt worse.

Look back at Caroline's last diagram. Consider the links between each of the areas:

Q *When Caroline began walking faster and ignored her symptoms – what impact might this behaviour have had on worsening how she felt?*

Q *What factors drove her to press on regardless?*

Q *What could she try to change in the future to make things better?*

SECTION 3: Completing your own thought investigation

Now you have an opportunity for yourself to play thought detective, by looking in detail at a specific time when you have felt worse.

Step 1: Think in detail about a specific time recently when you have felt worse

Think in detail:

Where am I?

What am I doing?

Consider:

The time: What time of day is it?

The place: Where am I?

The people: Who is present. Who am I with?

The events: What has been said?/What events have occurred?

Step 2: Identify your key thought: what went through your mind at this time?

Some people find it easy to be aware of their own thoughts. However, it is quite common for people to find that it can be quite hard to notice their thoughts to begin with.

The following questions can help you identify your thoughts. Were there any thoughts about:

- Yourself/how you are coping?

- The worst thing that could happen?
- How others see you?
- Your own body, behaviour or performance?
- Any painful **memories** from the past?
- Did you notice any **images** or pictures in your mind? (Images are an important type of thought and can have a powerful impact on how you feel).

With practice, most people find that a number of different thoughts may be present at times when they feel worse. *Choose the thought that is upsetting you the most*, your **key thought**.

Write any thoughts you noticed here:

Write down your key thought here:

Overall, how much did you believe the key thought at that time?

Make a cross on the line below to record how much you believed the thought.

Not at all believed — Completely believed

0% 50% 100%

Knowing how much you believe the thought is useful; later in the workbook you will have a chance to challenge your belief in the thought.

Step 3: Does the key thought show one of the unhelpful thinking styles?

Everyone notices extreme and unhelpful thoughts from time to time. These sorts of thoughts can backfire and worsen how you feel. They are often present at times when you are struggling. Such thoughts are described as unhelpful thinking styles. Read through the list and select those unhelpful thinking styles that were present.

Unhelpful thinking style	*Some typical thoughts*	*Tick if you thought like this at the time your mood altered*
Putting a negative slant on things (negative mental filter)		Am I focusing on the bad in situations?
	I see things through dark-tinted glasses	☐
	I see the glass as being half empty rather than half full	☐
	Whatever I've done in the week it's never enough to give me a sense of achievement	☐
	I tend to focus on the bad side of everyday situations	☐
Jump to the worst conclusion (catastrophising)		Am I jumping to the very worst conclusion?
	I tend to predict that the very worst outcome will happen	☐
	I often think that I will fail badly	☐
Having a gloomy view of the future (make negative predictions)		Am I making negative predictions about the future?
	I think that things will stay bad or get even worse	☐
	I tend to predict that things will go wrong	☐
	If one thing goes wrong I often predict that everything will go wrong	☐
	I'm always looking for the next thing to fail	☐
Putting myself down (bias against myself)		Am I being my own worst critic?
	I'm very self-critical	☐
	I overlook my strengths.	☐
	I see myself as not coping	☐
	I don't recognise my achievements	☐

Unhelpful thinking style	*Some typical thoughts*	*Tick if you thought like this at the time your mood altered*
Negative view about how others see me (mind-reading)		Am I second-guessing that others see me badly without actually checking if it's actually true?
	I mind-read what others think of me	☐
	I often think that others don't like me/think badly of me without evidence	☐
	Others don't believe that I'm ill	☐
Bearing all responsibility		Am I *taking unfair responsibility* for things that aren't really my fault/taking all the blame?
	I think I should take the blame if things go wrong	☐
	I feel guilty about things that are not really my fault	☐
	I think I'm responsible for everyone else	☐
Making extreme statements/rules		Am I using unhelpful *must/should/ought/got to* statements? (making extreme statements or setting impossible standards)?
	I use the words 'always' and 'never' a lot to summarise things	☐
	If one bad thing happens to me I often say 'Just typical' because it seems this always happens	☐
	I make myself a lot of 'must', 'should', 'ought' or 'got to' rules	☐

Choice point

If the thought doesn't show one of the unhelpful thinking styles then you can stop here. If so, look back at any other thoughts you noticed at the time – do any of them show an unhelpful thinking style? If so, they might be a good choice as a key thought.

Step 4: How does this key thought affect you?

Does it worsen how you *feel* and unhelpfully alter what you *do*?

1. The impact of the immediate thoughts on your emotions

Unhelpful thinking can unhelpfully change how you feel so that you may become disheartened, anxious, angry or demoralised.

What you think can worsen how you feel emotionally.

Unhelpful thinking ⟶ Worsened mood

What was the impact of the immediate thoughts on how you felt emotionally at the time?

Helpful ☐ Unhelpful ☐

2. The impact of the immediate thoughts on your behaviour

What you think can affect what you do.

Unhelpful thinking ⟶ Reduced/avoided activity or unhelpful behaviours

Consider the impact of your key thought on your behaviour and how this affected you and others.

Reduced activity		
Did it cause me to stop/reduce doing something	Yes ☐	No ☐
I was forced to rest and change my plans for the next few days	Yes ☐	No ☐
Avoidance		
Did it cause me to avoid any situations	Yes ☐	No ☐
Did it cause me to avoid talking to or meeting anyone	Yes ☐	No ☐
Did I avoid doing a planned activity as a result	Yes ☐	No ☐
Unhelpful behaviours: consider the impact on your symptoms, feelings and on your relationships in both the short and longer term		
I put 110 per cent of my energy into what I was doing	Yes ☐	No ☐
I kept asking for reassurance from others (e.g. family/friends/ internet chat room, etc.)	Yes ☐	No ☐
I was irritable and pushed people away	Yes ☐	No ☐
I stopped everything (e.g. went to bed and stayed there)	Yes ☐	No ☐
I did something that set me up to fail	Yes ☐	No ☐
I started checking myself over physically	Yes ☐	No ☐

I did something that set me up to be let down or rejected	Yes ☐	No ☐
I contacted the doctor/hospital when past experience told me I really didn't need to	Yes ☐	No ☐
I misused my tablets (e.g. by taking an extra dose that wasn't prescribed)	Yes ☐	No ☐
I had a drink to block how I felt or to help me relax	Yes ☐	No ☐
I looked up my symptoms on the internet/in a book	Yes ☐	No ☐
Other:		
Write any other altered behaviour you did here:		
What was the impact of the key thought on what you did at the time your mood altered?	Helpful ☐	Unhelpful ☐

Summary

Having answered these questions, what was the consequence of any altered behaviour you made?

- **Did reduced activity prevent you from doing something that you had planned to do?**
- **Did avoidance lead you to restrict your life or undermine your confidence?**
- **Did unhelpful behaviours end up backfiring or worsening how you or others feel?**
- **Finally, did believing the thought prevent you from doing something helpful – like going out/staying active?**

3. The impact of the immediate thoughts on your symptoms

Unhelpful thinking can make you focus more on your symptoms and can set off cycles of worry which make you feel worse.

What you think can worsen how you feel physically.

Unhelpful thinking ——→ Worsened symptoms

What was the impact of the key thought on your symptoms?

Helpful ☐ Unhelpful ☐ Unsure ☐

Overall, *did the key thought have an unhelpful effect on you?*

Yes ☐ No ☐

If you answered Yes to this question, go to **Step 5. Otherwise, keep reading!**

If a thought shows one of the unhelpful thinking styles, and also has an unhelpful impact on you, then you have identified an example of an extreme and unhelpful thought. These are the sorts of thoughts that you will learn to challenge in the next section ('Changing unhelpful thinking').

Step 5: Stop, think and reflect on the key thought

Simply noticing the key thought and becoming aware of its effects may be enough.

- **Try to label the key thought as *just another* of those extreme and unhelpful thoughts.** These are just a part of what happens to most people in times of upset.
- **Allow the thought to 'just be'.** Try to take a step back from the thought as if observing it from a distance. Move your mind on to other more helpful things such as the future or recent achievements.
- **Move on.** Make an active choice to stay active/face any unhelpful fears/choose to react helpfully rather than unhelpfully.

Summary of my thought investigation of a time when my mood changed

Now that you have finished, re-read your answers in your thought investigation.

The whole process is summarised in the Toolbox (p. 291).

REMEMBER

Sometimes people find that when they start noticing their thoughts, they end up thinking about them a lot of the time. If this is the case for you then allowing the thoughts just 'to be' is an important step.

Choice point

If the approach is helpful, then you can stop here. If you find you are still upset by the key thought, go to Section 4.

If you have decided to stop here it might be important to spend time being aware of any unhelpful thoughts you might have, before moving on. This could become your current goal for the next few days. If you intend to move on, you can set your goal at the end of the workbook.

My current goal

Perfectionism: the harsh task master

For many people with functional neurological symptoms, perfectionism and high standards are a key issue. You may have noticed already even in completing the workbooks that worries creep in about how well you are completing the tasks/ questions, etc.

There are many benefits to being someone with high standards:

- You may produce high-quality work.
- Others may admire the things you do and the standard of your work.
- Doing things well can be rewarding.

However, many people with very high standards can find that these backfire at times. This can be especially the case when they are struggling to cope because of their symptoms. For example:

- If you are driven by *should/must/ought* rules then you may have some immediate satisfaction on completing things. However, many people find that this is forgotten fairly quickly and then start looking for the next thing to do.
- Because there is a pressure to do things very well, the person may feel constantly stressed as they do their work. You can become worried by the thought of failure.
- Some tasks may take longer and require more effort as you constantly try to get things 'just right'. For example, painting a room can become a nightmare if every hair from the paintbrush has to be removed and every surface made absolutely smooth. It becomes impossible to enjoy things and feel a sense of achievement or pleasure in things as a result.
- The resulting behaviour can be frustrating for others. People with high standards can sometimes be frustrating to other people, and can even become annoying if they try to foist their standards onto everyone else.

This idea of high standards can also become a yardstick against which you judge yourself. If for example you find you struggle to achieve these standards then you can end up judging yourself as a failure. These sorts of black and white thoughts can make you feel as if you are not coping.

Look back at the example of Caroline on page 159. She overly pushes herself to meet goals that are unrealistic and unnecessary ('I must reach the turning point or I'll have failed'). You can find out ways of overcoming perfectionism in Section 4 of this workbook.

Some common difficulties

Some ways of dealing with unhelpful thoughts don't work.

1. Trying hard not to think about things

Because worrying thoughts focus on topics that are distressing you may try hard *not* to think about the thoughts. Remember your white polar bear – is this an effective strategy?

For many people, trying hard to ignore their upsetting thoughts and not think about them doesn't work and may actually worsen the problem. This can be mentally exhausting.

Do I end up putting a lot of mental effort into trying hard not to think the upsetting thoughts?

Yes ☐ No ☐

If I try not to think the thoughts, does it work?

Yes ☐ No ☐

2. Rumination: going over the same things again and again in your mind

A second common response is to try to think your way out of the situation by over-analysing any concerns in great detail. The result is that the same spirals of thoughts go round and round in your head. However, this approach also isn't usually effective. It is far more effective to just *let the thoughts be* and accept that you have these worries and that you cannot think your way through them.

3. Catastrophising – imagining the very worst

It is common to develop fears about your symptoms and how they might make you look or behave in public. For example, you can worry about looking odd, falling over or dropping something. It is important to remember that sometimes these things may actually happen but they are not necessarily as catastrophic as you imagine them to be. Therefore it's really important not to let the catastrophic thoughts you have limit what you do.

Misinterpretation of symptoms

Sometimes people can become overly sensitive to illness and misinterpret everyday symptoms as being evidence of serious disease. For example, someone like Patrick who has heart disease may pay special attention to quite normal variations in his heart rate. He becomes scared of doing things that raise his heart rate just in case it is dangerous. This is not to say that someone in that situation should exercise a lot. However, it raises the possibility that you can sometimes be overly protective of yourself. To make a decision about the **right balance** of activity, seek clear advice from doctors and healthcare practitioners that is based on their professional assessment of your current physical state. Problems arise when people either ignore this and overdo things, or become overly aware of illness and avoid doing anything at all.

How does this situation arise?

We've already discussed this in Workbook 3 but it will be helpful to read the explanation again. Have you changed where you live recently or do you know of anyone who has? Think about that experience. As someone looks to buy or rent a flat or house, they suddenly begin to notice that there are a lot of houses advertised wherever they go. Similarly when someone changes their car they find that everyone is now driving the same model! The key point is that you become very aware of things that are relevent to you at the time. This applies to flats, houses and cars. It also applies to physical health symptoms and health-related information. When people are worried about illness and its consequences, they tend to watch out for information or symptoms that are relevant to them. This especially applies to anything that might feel threatening or scary.

For example, if you have rheumatoid arthritis, you are more likely to pay attention to newspaper or television reports about new treatments of this disease. The same principle applies to how you scan and pay special attention to particular scary physical symptoms that seem particularly threatening. Patrick has had a previous heart attack. He is therefore more likely to pay special attention to the speed of his pulse, and to any twinges of pain in his chest – whatever the cause. Of course in moderation this is sensible, however, it can backfire if it leads him to become so anxious about his pulse that he is taking it all the time. When taken to such an extreme extent, Patrick may find that he is unable to do any exercise at all, even though physically it might be completely safe (and actually recommended as part of his heart recovery programme).

These responses occur in everyone. For example:

- Large screening programs by occupational health departments often pick up possible problems such as high blood pressure (hypertension) or abnormal ECG heart tracing results. Those people are then referred on for a specialist assessment 'just to be sure'. Most of those people are then given a clean bill of health. However, in spite of this they are more likely to feel unwell than before the tests were done in the first place. The health 'scare' has upset them. Even though they are not ill, they feel worse than before.

- Medical students often visit the doctor with health concerns about the area of health that they are studying at the time. For example, they are more prone to present with bowel symptoms shortly after learning about all the different diseases that affect the bowel.

This process of selectively focusing on symptoms and misinterpreting normal sensations as signs of illness can occur in everyone. The two examples show how common milder health anxieties are. The health fears usually fall away quite quickly over a period of weeks or months. Health fears can occur alongside physical disease or in its absence. The latter situation is called **health anxiety**. Section 4 deals with this in more detail, including using thought investigation.

KEY POINT

Noticing changes in how you feel can be a helpful way of identifying extreme and unhelpful thinking.

If a thought shows one or more of the unhelpful thinking styles, and has an unhelpful impact on how you feel or what you do, then you have identified an example of an extreme and an unhelpful thought. These are the sort of thoughts that will be the focus for change in the next section of the workbook.

With regular use you may come to realise that even in different situations you tend to have the same style of unhelpful thoughts. You can learn more about this in the next section.

In Section 4, you will learn about how to begin to challenge extreme and unhelpful thinking. For the time being, try to get used to carrying out a thought investigation. There is a blank Five Areas assessment diagram in Toolbox E, on page 292, for you to photocopy and use as many times as you like. Once you feel confident in doing this, you should move on to the next section on changing unhelpful thinking.

SECTION 4: Changing unhelpful thinking

The following skills aim to help you to begin questioning the stream of extreme and unhelpful thoughts that 'pop' into the mind through the day. In times when you feel worse, these unhelpful thinking styles come to mind more often than usual, and are more likely to be believed.

Examples of extreme and unhelpful thoughts include:

- 'I'm going to have to rest or I will make myself worse.'
- 'I'll never get better.'
- 'It's been a terrible week.'
- 'If I don't sit down now, I will fall over.'
- 'Nothing I do is going to make any difference to this.'
- 'Here we go again. If my headache is here, my other symptoms are sure to follow.'
- 'I should just be able to put all this behind me and return to normal.'

At the moment it is likely that when you notice thoughts like these you often tend to accept that they are true. You may notice that they are easier to believe when you feel worse.

One effective way to improve how you feel is to practise skills of how to challenge these thoughts. As you become better at this, you will find you are able to challenge the thoughts at more difficult times.

You have already practised how to identify extreme and unhelpful key thoughts in Section 2 of the workbook. The next stage is to use a three-point plan to bring about change:

1 **Question** the helpfulness and accuracy of the key thought(s).

2 Come to a **balanced conclusion** about the key thought(s).

3 Experiment: **Apply** the balanced conclusion to what you do.

This thought challenge approach of **identify, question, conclude and apply** can help you begin to change unhelpful thinking.

KEY POINT

Don't choose thoughts like 'I am …', 'People are …' or 'The world is …' for the time being as these thoughts are harder to tackle at first.

So how could things be different?

Initially it looks like Caroline could do nothing to change the situation. But, as you saw in Section 1, how people think can really make a difference to what happens. Looking more closely at her thought investigation, if Caroline could have changed her key thought this might have affected her behaviour, symptoms and feelings.

Imagine if she had been kinder to herself and hadn't been driven on by her should/must/ought rules she may have set herself an easier target or allowed herself to stop and rest. By doing this her symptoms might not have become so extreme and she would have been less upset. Choosing to take control over such a distressing situation can boost confidence and create a sense of achievement. This may seem straightforward but can take time to master in practice. You will learn more about how to do this in the rest of this workbook.

This **thought flashcard** has been designed to help you to practise this process of carrying out a thought investigation whenever you feel worse. The thought flashcard is available in Toolbox E (p. 293).

Getting the most from the thought flashcard of a time when you feel worse.

★ With practice you will find it easier to identify your own extreme and unhelpful thinking.

★ Try to fill the flashcard in as soon as possible after you notice the change.

★ If you cannot fill it in immediately, try to think yourself back into the situation so that you are as clear as possible in your answer.

Step 6: Reflect on the key thought in more detail

It's easy to believe the worst when people are upset.

Question the thought – don't just accept it. For example, is there anything to make Caroline think her key thought 'I must get to the turning point or I'll have failed' is incorrect?

You might find it helpful to imagine you are in a courtroom demanding answers of the thought. Here is how Caroline did it.

Example

Why did I have to get to the turning point at all costs?

If I hadn't got there would that have made me a failure?

Caroline uses the **seven key thought challenge questions** – the questions the key thought doesn't want her to ask:

- What would I tell a friend who said the same thing?

Example

I'd tell her that she does so well keeping on top of her symptoms and keeping the house and family running – that getting to a turning point isn't so important.

- If I wasn't feeling like this what would I say?

Example

I'd say that not doing something 100 per cent doesn't make me a failure.

- Am I basing this on how I feel rather than the facts?

Example

Yes, because even going for a walk every day is something I wasn't able to do a year ago.

- What would other people say? Have I heard different opinions from others about the same thought?

Example

Everyone close to me, especially my husband says I do a great job; no one has told me I'm a failure.

- Am I looking at the whole picture? Are there any other ways of explaining the situation that are more accurate?

Example

I discounted the bits of the day that were ok, like getting the kids to school and enjoying the start of the walk.

- What would I say about this looking back in six months time?

Example

Why did you let a small thing like not walking exactly your usual route ruin your whole day?

- Do I apply one set of standards to myself and another to others?

Definitely.

In the same way, you may find it helpful to come up with a new balanced and helpful conclusion based upon your answers to these questions. Caroline's is given below.

Example: Caroline's balanced conclusion

If I hadn't got to the turning point it wouldn't have made me a failure and if I'd stopped earlier I might not have ended up in bed in the afternoon.

Re-rate your belief in the key thought

Not at all — × 80% — Completely believed

0% — 100%

If you find this approach helpful, then you can stop here. But if are you still upset by the thought go to step 7. Caroline decides to move on to step 7.

Step 7: Experiment: act against the original key thought

It is important to decide not to be pushed around by the unhelpful thought. A good way of doing this is:

1 **Let it be** – choose not to turn it over again and again.

Example

I just need to move on and put today behind me.

2 Choose to **act against** the unhelpful thought. For example, if the thought says to you 'Don't go to the meal, you won't enjoy it' – then go to the meal. If it says to you 'Nobody wants to talk to you' – then choose to talk to someone and see how they react. If it says 'You can only cope if you stay in bed or stop all activities' then choose not to stay in bed and stop everything – but instead respond more helpfully.

One powerful action you can do to test the helpfulness and accuracy of the balanced conclusion is to **act on the balanced conclusion**, believing it to be true, and see what happens. This may mean choosing to do the *reverse* of what the immediate thought may be telling you. What test (s) could Caroline set up? Look at her plan below.

Example: Caroline's plan for putting her balanced conclusion into practice

I'll make a list of the reasons why I'm not a failure and keep it with me in case this thought comes back. I could also ask other people, friends and family the type of person they think is a failure.

Example

The next time I go for a walk I won't set myself a target of getting to my usual turning point; instead I'll make a point of enjoying my walk, looking at the scenery in the park and I'll remind myself of my achievements. Having definite set in stone targets just sets me up to fail.

KEY POINT

By far the best evidence for or against a thought is found through looking at the consequences of what happens when you choose to act or not act on it. Reinforce your balanced conclusions by acting on them. Undermine your extreme and unhelpful thoughts by acting against them.

Experiment: putting the balanced conclusion into practice

You are asked to a party. Your initial reaction is to say no as a result of an immediate thought: 'I won't enjoy it'. Try to act against this thought (by going to the party) in order to test out whether it is true. You may well find that the party goes better than you predicted and that you do enjoy it at least a little.

Write your plans here:

To undermine the immediate extreme and unhelpful thought:

To reinforce my new balanced conclusion:

Have I created a plan to put my balanced conclusion into practice?

Yes ☐ No ☐

Note: It may take time to build your confidence in this. The workbooks on overcoming avoidance, reduced activity and unhelpful behaviours may help you plan ways of slowly making these changes at a pace that you can cope with.

KEY POINT

Acting against your extreme and unhelpful thoughts will help undermine them.

The impact of balanced thoughts

The purpose of showing you Caroline's example was to try to illustrate the process of challenging extreme and unhelpful thoughts. By asking the series of questions, Caroline was able to begin to produce an alternative conclusion that was:

1 Helpful.

2 More balanced and true.

And she was able to change what she did (her behaviour) as a result.

You will now have the opportunity to practise these skills for yourself on one of your own extreme and unhelpful thoughts.

SECTION 5: Practice changing my key thought

Step 6: Reflect on the key thought in more detail

It's easy to believe the worst when you are upset. Look back to page 163 to identify your key thought.

Question the thought – don't just accept it. Is there anything to make you think the key thought is incorrect? You might find it helpful to imagine you are in a courtroom demanding answers of the thought. Write in your own answers to these questions here:

Use the seven key thought challenge questions – the questions the key thought doesn't want you to ask:

- What would I tell a friend who said the same thing?

- If I wasn't feeling like this what would I say?

- Am I basing this on how I feel rather than the facts?

- What would other people say? Have I heard different opinions from others about the same thought?

- Am I looking at the whole picture? Are there any other ways of explaining the situation that are more accurate?

- What would I say about this looking back in six months time?

- Do I apply one set of standards to myself and another to others?

You may find it helpful to come up with a new **balanced and helpful conclusion** based upon your answers to these questions.

My balanced conclusion:

Like a celebrity, key thoughts love attention. It's just not worth your attention. Allow it to *just be*.

Re-rate your belief in the key thought

Not at all (0%)	______________________________	Completely believed (100%)

The series of questions that you have answered have helped you to *stop, think and reflect* on your immediate thought in a structured way. Look at the rating of the amount you believe the immediate extreme and unhelpful thought *before and after* this questioning process. If the amount you believe the original extreme thought has dropped, this is a sign that you have been able (at least in part) to challenge the thought.

If this proved difficult, don't give up. It takes time to learn how to effectively question and challenge extreme and unhelpful thoughts. It may be difficult at first to break the habit of extreme and unhelpful thinking, particularly if you have been coping with symptoms for some time. Keep trying though, and you will find that it becomes easier.

If this approach helps, then you can stop here. If you find you are still upset by the thought go to step 7.

Step 7: Experiment: act against the original key thought

It is important to decide not to be pushed around by the negative thought. A good way of doing this is:

1 *Let it be* – choose not to turn it over again and again.

2 Choose to *act against* the unhelpful thought.

Putting the balanced conclusion into practice

One helpful approach to find out whether the new balanced conclusion is true and helpful is to **set up a test** to see if it is true in practice. Having already looked at Caroline's example, what test(s) could you set up?

One powerful action you can do to test the helpfulness and accuracy of the balanced conclusion is to **act on the balanced conclusion**, believing it to be true, and see what happens. This may mean choosing to do the **reverse** of what the immediate thought may be telling you.

> KEY POINT
>
> **By far the best evidence for or against a thought is found through looking at the consequences of what happens when you choose to act or not act on it. Reinforce your balanced conclusions by acting on them. Undermine your extreme and unhelpful thoughts by acting against them.**

My plan for putting my balanced conclusion into practice

1 To undermine the immediate extreme and unhelpful thought:

2 To reinforce my new balanced conclusion:

Have you created a **plan** to put your balanced conclusion into practice?

Yes ☐ No ☐

Summary

The questions you have worked through can be applied to any extreme and unhelpful thoughts that result in you feeling worse. By examining, questioning and challenging these thoughts, you will begin to change the way you see yourself, your current situation and the future.

KEY POINTS

- **Begin to pay attention to, and to challenge, any extreme and unhelpful thoughts.**
- **Your extreme and unhelpful thoughts will slowly change as you begin to challenge them in a regular way. By continuing to do this, you will develop more balanced, moderate and helpful thinking.**

A thought flashcard, which brings together all the steps you have practised in this workbook, has been developed to allow you to practise identifying and then challenging extreme and unhelpful thoughts. You will find the flashcard in Toolbox E, page 293. You can tear this out or photocopy it if you wish, along with the Five Areas assessment diagram. Try to carry these around with you in order to help you to identify and challenge any extreme and unhelpful thoughts. With practice, you will find that it becomes easier to do this and you will be able to develop more balanced, moderate and helpful thinking. You can also download it for free from www.fiveareas.com.

Other helpful things to try

Don't let your thoughts push you around

Letting yourself be pushed around by worrying thoughts reduces anxiety in the short term but it just keeps them coming back. In fact, the more attention you give them, the more they return. However, if you find ways to resist them you find that they become less important. You can even increase your self-confidence through resisting them.

This might sound a bit simple, however if it were that simple you would have already stopped worrying. It's important not to feel too defeated; worrying thoughts squeeze out any helpful thoughts and you forget that you have coped with difficult situations in the past. Once a period of acute stress and worry is over you should go through the thought challenge worksheet and try to question the thought. In the beginning, it's important to do this when you feel less stressed as worrying thoughts crowd out everything else. The more you practise the quicker and easier this will become.

Perfectionism: go for grey

You might be someone who has always believed, no matter how well you've done, that you could have done better. This results in the feeling of always having failed or never being quite *good enough*. To overcome these black and white thinking styles you need to try to aim for shades of grey. For example, as you saw with Caroline if her goal had been different she could have deemed her walk a success. Naz has struggled to change his perfectionist ideas, he believed that being a young man but being unable to play football made him a failure. When he made a conscious decision to get back to football in small, planned steps he found he could.

It might be helpful for you to weigh up the advantages and disadvantages of perfectionism if these affect you. It can be useful to write these down in two columns on a blank piece of paper. If you find it hard to be objective ask someone who knows you well to help.

Perfectionism can also stop you getting started on things because you fear you won't meet your very high standards, so find it easier just not to start. If this type of perfectionism has affected you in the past, or is currently an issue, then think about how helpful this avoidance was. Having very high standards places undue stress on you, and perfectionists usually find that the harder they try, the more their disappointment increases.

Let upsetting thoughts 'just be'

To help you allow the thoughts to 'just be' try to actively bring on the unsettling thought *more than usual*. Instead of trying hard not to think it, do the reverse. Deliberately bring on the thought again and again. To help you do this, try the following:

- Write it down in detail again and again, thinking about it as you do so.
- Speak out the thought in great detail, describing what would occur if the worst were to happen. Consider recording this and playing it back again and again. Pay attention to what you think and feel. Saying the thought or fear will not cause it to occur.
- As you do so, be aware of any attempts to neutralise or 'make good' the thought, such as making promises to yourself. Try to increase this for increasing lengths of time.

- The purpose of doing this is to realise that having the thought does not cause the distressing events to occur. The thought is not as powerful as you think it is.

Eventually by doing this you will find that the thought makes you feel less and less upset, and that these feelings last for shorter and shorter periods of time. *Try to aim to spend so much time with the thought that you become bored by it.* The aim is to be able to say to yourself, 'It's just another of those extreme and unhelpful thoughts again.' Notice it as if from a distance and then carry on with life.

A key target is therefore for you to aim to *get used* to the thoughts and *become less stressed* about them. To illustrate this, imagine if a large bluebottle was in the same room as you. If you run around trying unsuccessfully to catch it, this will only make it more excited so that it buzzes around even more noisily than before. Sometimes the best approach is just to ignore it and allow it to be. Although this does not remove the bluebottle from the room, it causes a lot less problems. This is most successful in overcoming this pattern of over-thinking. In the same way, if you notice that you tend to go over things again and again in your mind:

- Break the cycle – choose not to keep thinking the same old thoughts.
- Again just allow the thoughts to be – with time they will lose their power.

Core beliefs

Everyone has core beliefs; they are how you make sense of the world and yourself. They provide you with a shortcut in daily life. Imagine chatting to someone at a social event and finding it quite awkward. This might trigger the core belief 'Nobody likes me' and use the difficult conversation as instant evidence to support this. It is a much quicker way to make sense of the situation than to think through all the possibilities of why this might be uncomfortable. It could be something to do with the other person; for example, they may be tired, not very good at meeting new people or be distracted by their own worries. Core beliefs can make us very critical of ourselves. You often wouldn't be as judgemental about your worst enemy as you are about yourself.

How to spot that the thought you're trying to challenge might be a core belief

If you find a recurrent theme that underlies lots of your unhelpful thoughts, it is likely to be a core belief. They don't just occur in relation to one situation or topic, they pop up lots of times and will have done so throughout your life, maybe without you realising. For example, Caroline felt a failure for not reaching the turning point. She also remembered feeling the same way in the past when she was in bed for several weeks. In fact, when Caroline really thought about it, she realised that since her early teens she'd had similar thoughts about loads of different situations and life events. Even when she got a good job she felt she should have had a job like that at a much younger age.

Core beliefs are not necessarily true but are very strong. They usually develop when you are young and learning about the world and yourself. Caroline realises that she often thinks of herself as a failure. She can relate this to when she was growing up. Her older sister was exceptionally clever and also very sporty. Caroline grew up believing that she would never be as good at anything as her sister. This led her to ignore all the great things she did and consider herself a failure. Her core belief is that she's a failure and has to try twice as hard as everyone else to be successful. As is common with core beliefs, other people would not see things the same way as Caroline. They would never judge her to be a failure and, in fact, would be surprised to find that she thought this way.

KEY POINT

Core beliefs are your own very judgemental thoughts and they often don't reflect reality.

Core beliefs are more difficult to challenge than other thoughts. If you think you've found a core belief then you've done well to identify it and you can begin to question how helpful this belief is to you in your life.

Techniques to challenge core beliefs

Usually to really get to challenge core beliefs you need to seek out a longer-term course of expert delivered cognitive behavioural therapy (CBT). A list of accredited CBT practitioners in the UK is available at www.babcp.com. The sort of work done to alter core beliefs includes keeping a diary of evidence against your core belief and weighing up the evidence gathered objectively. For example, Caroline easily overlooked her success as a mother and other areas of her life when viewing herself as a complete failure for not reaching the turning point.

You can also repeatedly question how helpful it has been in your life to hold a particular belief, and write down your answers. Usually people find that holding a particular core belief has been unhelpful at least sometimes in the past. At this point creating a less extreme belief and testing out what others think can be useful. At the end of completing these sorts of exercises some people might still have the thought 'I know all that but it still feels true'. These are beliefs that have been with people for a long time and usually take time and work to change. Here, working with a CBT specialist can be helpful. However, even raising your own awareness of the impact these beliefs can have on your life can be helpful.

SECTION 6: Summary

In this workbook you have:

- **Briefly reviewed how your thought investigation and thought change practice went.**
- **Learned and practised how to challenge extreme and unhelpful thoughts.**
- **Developed balanced conclusions and created plans to put them into practice.**

Putting into practice what you have learned

You have already begun to identify important changes in what you think and do. To build on this use the two sides of the **thought flashcards** to help you go through the process of **identifying, questioning and challenging** extreme and unhelpful thoughts on *four* occasions when your mood alters during the next week.

If you have difficulties with this, don't worry. Just do what you can and discuss any problems with your healthcare practitioner.

Once you have completed several flashcards over the next week, it is advisable to continue practising this approach using the flashcards as prompts over a number of weeks. With practice you will find that you become skilled at using this approach, and can begin to identify and challenge extreme thoughts without the help of the worksheet.

My current goal

How will you build on what you have learnt in this workbook?

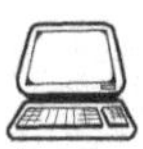

You can get additional help and support in problem solving at www.livinglifetothefull.com

Acknowledgements

The use of the Five Areas assessment model and associated language is used from the Overcoming Five Areas series by permission of Hodder Arnold Publishers and Dr C Williams. Illustrations are by Keith Chan and are reproduced by permission.

My notes

Part 3

Practical Toolboxes

The information in this section is aimed at giving you practical skills to put into practice in your own life.

Contents

The thought investigation flashcard and a blank Five Areas assessment sheet are given at the end of Toolbox E.

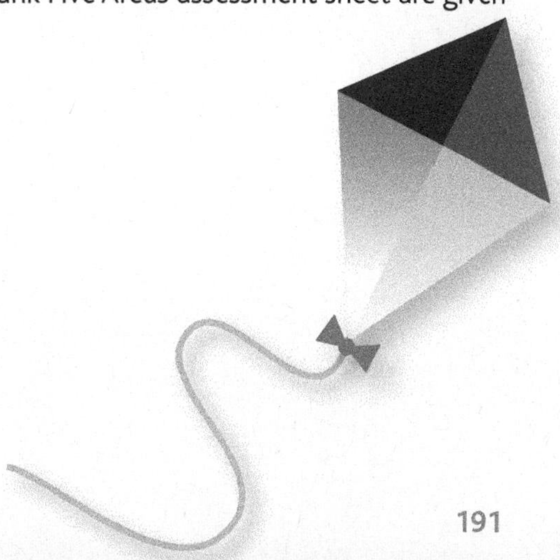

Toolbox A

Overcoming reduced activity and avoidance

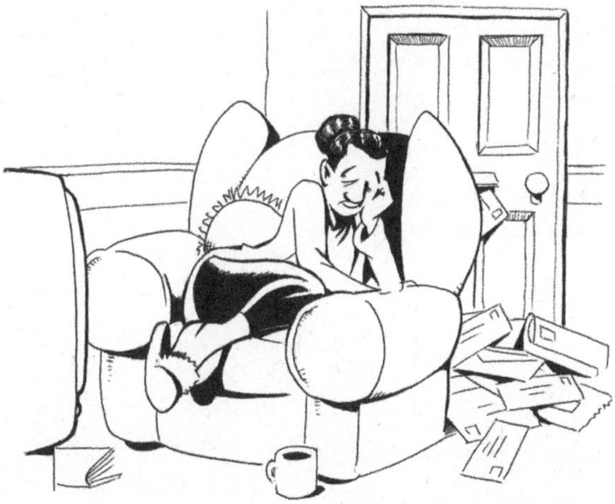

overcoming

functional neurological symptoms:
A Five Areas Approach

SECTION 1: Creating your own plan to increase your activity levels or overcome avoidance

You have read in Workbook 4 about how to plan to overcome reduced activity and avoidance. This section will help you to put what you have learned into action in your own life.

> STARTING OUT
>
> **If it has been some time since you read Workbook 4, and you may find it helpful to quickly look back through it now.**

In Workbook 4 you answered questions summarising activities that are commonly altered when you are coping with symptoms. This helped you to identify your **vicious circle of reduced activity**.

Keeping an activity diary to record your different activities

To find out to what extent the symptoms are affecting what you do, the first step is to begin to keep an activity diary for a week.

> KEY POINT
>
> **It is very important when completing the activity diary to watch out for negative thoughts that may cause you to discount or overlook your achievements. For someone who is facing the challenge of symptoms, the act of getting up and getting dressed can be a very large achievement. Symptoms such as a lack of energy and tiredness can interfere significantly with your ability to carry out activities most people do automatically (e.g. getting dressed). It is easy when feeling like this to think: 'Well, I should do that anyway/anyone could do that' and downplay your achievements. Try to look out for these negative thoughts and *write down what you did anyway*.**

The purpose of this is to allow you to gather information to help you to understand how your symptoms affect you. This will allow you to plan specific changes to your life. Most people need to practise gathering this information for a week or two to begin to work out the relationship between the activity and how they feel.

The aim is to help you to:

- **Understand links between your activities and how you feel.**
- **Discover if any specific activities or specific situations are linked to feeling better or worse.**

The diary can also be used to plan changes in what you do to:

- Combat inactivity.
- Increase pleasure in the activities you do.
- Recognise your achievements.
- Plan to do some of the activities that you previously enjoyed but which you have reduced or stopped or avoided because of your symptoms.

This approach will allow you to plan in advance what you are going to do each day. The aim is to increase specific activity levels to boost your feelings of pleasure and sense of achievement.

KEY POINT

We are not aiming to increase your total activity across the board. Instead the plan is to slowly increase *specific* activities that you have noticed give you a sense of pleasure or achievement. It may be that the thought of re-starting or increasing some of these activities seems daunting or impossible. The key is to use a step-by step plan where no step seems too large. Initially using this approach may result in you doing less overall than you are at the moment, but then you will gradually increase the amount you do.

Rate *each* activity you do for:

1 **Pleasure** (0–10 scale) experienced

2 How much of an **achievement** (0–10 scale) was this, based on how you feel now?

Scale

0	5	10
No pleasure/ achievement	Feel okay/ reasonable	Complete pleasure/ achievement

Bear in mind how your symptoms are currently affecting your ability to do things. How much of an achievement was doing the activity? Try to be fair in how you judge this.

What activities should I record?

Use the activity diary to record everything that you do over the next week. This might include:

- Getting dressed.
- Talking to a friend on the phone.
- Doing some housework, going out shopping, washing your hair, doing the washing-up.
- Also include times when you are sitting and watching television, having a bath or resting, etc.

On the next two pages are activity diaries that you can fill in. The first is a detailed diary for a whole day. The second is similar but covers a whole week. Some people prefer to use the first type while others prefer the second. It really doesn't matter which one you use as long as you remember to write down your pleasure and achievement scores for each activity. You might like to start by using the daily diary and then switch to the weekly one when you have got used to it – or you can make copies of the daily diary and keep using it for the whole week.

My daily activity diary

Day and date	*Activity (include everything you do)*	*Duration (how long did you do it for?)*	*Pleasure*	*Achievement*
7–8 am				
8–9 am				
9–10 am				
10–11 am				
11–12 am				
12–1 pm				
1–2 pm				
2–3 pm				
3–4 pm				
4–5 pm				
6–7 pm				
7–8 pm				
8–9 pm				
9–10 pm				
10–11 pm				

Achievement (A)

How much of an achievement was it, given how you feel?

0 = no sense of achievement.

5 = reasonable achievement.

10 = maximum sense of achievement.

Pleasure (P)

0 = no pleasure.

5 = feel okay.

10 = maximum pleasure.

My weekly activity diary

	Monday		Tuesday		Wednesday		Thursday		Friday		Saturday		Sunday	
	Activity	P/A	Activity	P/A	Activity	P/A	Activity	P/A	Activity	P/A	Activity	P/A	Activity	P/A
6 am														
7 am														
8 am														
9 am														
10 am														
11 am														
12 pm														
1 pm														
2 pm														
3 pm														
4 pm														
5 pm														
6 pm														
7 pm														
8 pm														
9 pm														
10 pm														

Reflect on your diary

How much pleasure do you experience during the day?

Does what you do seem to affect how you feel?

Do you get pleasure and a sense of achievement from the same things?

In particular, what things do you do that boost how you feel? For example, what impact does spending time and feeling close to people have?

Are there things missing from your diary that you used to do and are now avoiding because of symptoms or over-worry?

Now that you have gathered this background information, you can move on to use the following seven-step plan to map out the very first thing to change.

SECTION 2: The seven-step plan

Step 1: Identify the activity to build upon or problem area of avoidance to overcome

Look back through your activity diaries for the week. The important next step is to identify an **initial target area** that is *clearly defined*. This step is particularly important if you feel overwhelmed by several different problems. In doing this, it is important that you choose a target problem that:

1 Will be *useful* for changing how you are.

2 Is a *specific* target problem so that you will know when you have done it.

3 Is *realistic*: it is practical and achievable.

Select only *one target area* that you wish to change at the present time.

My **initial** target area is:

Is this a clear, focused target for change?

Yes ☐ No ☐

Will it be useful for understanding or changing how you are?

Yes ☐ No ☐

Is it a **specific task** *so that you will know when you have done it?*

Yes ☐ No ☐

Is it **realistic**: *is it practical and achievable for you?*

Yes ☐ No ☐

You should have been able to answer 'Yes' to all four questions. If you didn't, please go back and re-write your plan to tackle this.

Step 2: Think up as many solutions as possible to plan this next step

You now need to bridge the gap between what you do now and what you would like to do. You can bridge this gap by planning to do your activity in a number of *small* steps. You should identify a **single first step** to change that is *clearly defined* and which you want to do.

Try to come up with as many different things you could do to fulfil this first step. Useful questions to help you to think up possible solutions include:

- What *ridiculous* solutions can I include as well as more sensible ones?
- What helpful ideas would others (e.g. family, friends or colleagues at work) suggest?
- What approaches have I tried in the past in similar circumstances?
- What advice would I give a friend who was trying to tackle the same problem?

Write your solutions below:

Step 3: Look at the advantages and disadvantages of each of the possible activities

Assess how effective and practical each potential solution or chosen activity is. This involves considering the advantages and disadvantages for each of your potential solutions (the *pros* and *cons* of each possible option). Add additional boxes if you need them.

Suggestion	*Advantages*	*Disadvantages*

Step 4: Choose one of the solutions

Decide on a solution, based on what you have thought about in step 3.

This solution should be an option that lets you answer 'Yes' to the following two questions:

Is it helpful?

Yes ☐ No ☐

Is it achievable?

Yes ☐ No ☐

Step 5: Plan the steps needed to carry it out

My plan

Write your plan down here. Your task is to carry this out during the next week. Be mindful of anything that could possibly go wrong and plan for this too.

Check your plan against each of the questions for effective change.

The questions for effective change

Is the planned activity one that:

Is **useful** *for understanding or changing how I am?*

Yes ☐ No ☐

Is a **specific task** *so that I will know when I have done it?*

Yes ☐ No ☐

Is **realistic***: is it practical and achievable?*

Yes ☐ No ☐

*Makes clear **what** I am going to do and **when** I am going to do it?*

Yes ☐ No ☐

Is an activity that won't be easily blocked or prevented by practical problems?

Yes ☐ No ☐

You should have been able to answer *Yes* to each of the questions. If you have answered 'No' to one the questions, try to think why this is. What changes can you make to alter or improve your plan? Try to change or alter the activity so that any poorly planned aspects are improved.

Many people find this approach takes quite a lot of practice. It may also be tempting to be too ambitious. Before moving on, ask yourself again whether this is a target activity that you *really* can cope with at present. If not, change it for a more realistic target. Remember, large changes can be achieved by taking many little steps. There is an old Chinese proverb: 'A journey of a thousand miles begins with the first step ...' Do not push yourself too hard by being overly ambitious as this is only likely to set you up to fail.

When you can answer 'Yes' to each of the five questions above, it means that your activity is well planned out. Try to write down *exactly* what you will do and plan to put it into practice this week.

REMEMBER

Large changes can be achieved by moving one step at a time.

SECTION 3: Carrying out the plan and reflecting on it

Step 6: Carry out the plan

Remember that as you carry out the plan you are undermining your old fears by acting against them.

Put what you have planned into action.

Task

Write down any extreme and unhelpful thoughts you notice while carrying out your plan. Record how much you believe them at the time (from 0 – not at all, to 100 – believing them fully).

My fearful thought(s):

I believe this: ______ per cent **before** the task.

______per cent **during** the task.

______ per cent **after** the task.

Task

Record how anxious, worried or stressed you feel at the time (from 0 – no anxiety, stress or worry at all, to 100 the maximum anxiety, worry, stress possible).

My level of anxiety: ______ per cent **before** the task.

______per cent **during** the task.

______per cent **after** the task.

Step 7: Review the outcome

What happened when you carried out your plan? Try to pay attention to your thoughts about what would happen before, during and after you have completed the activity.

Write what happened here:

My review

Was the selected approach successful?

Yes ☐ No ☐

Did it help me to tackle the target problem?

Yes ☐ No ☐

Were there any disadvantages to using this approach?

Yes ☐ No ☐

What have I learned from what happened? Write in below:

When you have completed your planned activity, *look back and think about it*. Think in detail about how your planned activity went:

How much of a sense of achievement did you feel while doing the task?

Very little ———————————————— Very much

- If you noticed that the activity gave you a *high* sense of achievement at the time:

This is important because it shows that by altering your activity, you can also alter your sense of achievement in things. This can provide a powerful tool for overcoming health problems. Your experience also shows that you have picked an effective activity to change because it led to this feeling.

- If you noticed that the activity gave you *only a slight* sense of achievement at the time:

Try to think about the factors that robbed you of a higher sense of achievement at the time. Were you aware of any negative or undermining thoughts such as 'I *should* have done it anyway' or 'It's a waste of time'? You can learn how to identify and challenge unhelpful thoughts like these in Workbook 5. In the meantime, if thoughts such as these are present, try to *stop, think and reflect* on them rather than immediately accepting them as being true.

How much of a sense of pleasure did you experience while doing the task?

Very little ——————————————————————— Very much

- If you noticed that the activity gave you a *high* sense of pleasure at the time:

This shows that by altering your activity you can improve how you feel. Trying to increase your activity levels in this area in a step-by-step way may be helpful in improving how you feel.

- If you noticed that the activity gave you *only a slight* sense of pleasure at the time:

Try to think about the factors that prevented you from experiencing pleasure. Were you aware of any negative thoughts that undermined how you felt? Were you distracted by other concerns and therefore didn't allow yourself to stop, think and reflect on what you were doing? Sometimes, extreme and unhelpful statements or rules (such as *should, must, got to* and *ought*) may come into mind and undermine a person's pleasure in things. Did this happen to you?

HINT

Thinking back on the areas in the week that have been pleasurable can act to boost how you feel. Look back on your activity diary and record positive events such as conversations, activities, etc. that have provided you with a sense of pleasure or achievement. Use this approach to try to develop a more helpful focus to your thinking as well as to help plan your activities. Build in a time each day to reflect on these events and remember positive aspects such as times when you feel close to others.

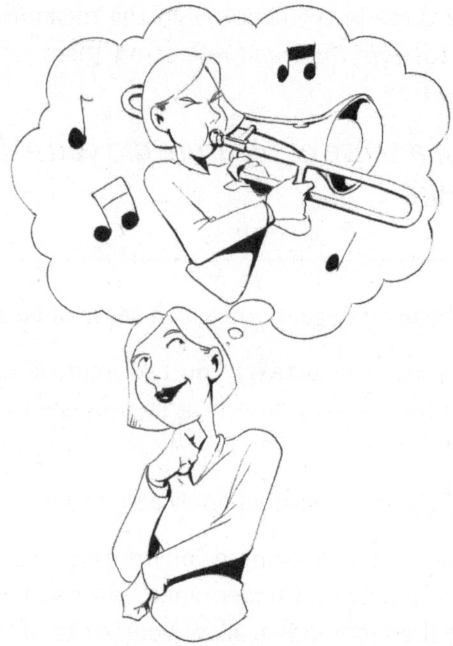

This idea of choosing to build in a **helpful focus** to at least part of your day can help improve how you feel. Try this approach to see if it is helpful for you. Decide to keep thinking from time to time about your achievements and take pleasure in what you have done.

Think again about how your target activity went:

How easy was it for you to do the task?

- If it was *fairly easy* for you to do the task:

This shows that you chose to do an activity that you could successfully complete. Choosing realistic targets for change is important. Choosing activities that are focused and clear, and which you can succeed in, is the key to effective change. Sometimes an activity can seem too easy. If this is the case, you have the option of choosing something that is a little harder next time. By making slow, sure steps you will be able to build your confidence and increase the things you do which give you a sense of pleasure and achievement.

- If it was *quite hard* for you to do the task:

Choosing realistic targets for change is important. Sometimes it is tempting to choose an activity that is too ambitious. Instead, choose activities that are focused and clear, and which you can succeed in. By making slow, sure steps you will be able to build your confidence and increase the things you do which give you a sense of pleasure and achievement. Applying the questions for effective change can help you to create a realistic action plan.

Did any problems or difficulties occur in what you did?

Yes ☐ No ☐

- If you had *some difficulties* in carrying out your planned activity:

This provides you with the opportunity to learn useful information for next time you plan an activity. Try to think about what happened. Could you have predicted the problem? What could you have done to prevent it? How could you put what you have learned into practice next time? Sometimes problems are unpredictable. If so, don't let yourself be put off trying this approach. Try it again. Use the problem as an opportunity to learn.

- If you *didn't have any difficulties* in carrying out your planned activity:

It is good if there were no difficulties in carrying out your activity. It is likely that you had planned it well.

Before planning any activity, it is important to consider whether it is realistic, and also to try to predict any possible blocks or difficulties. At some time when you do an activity, something may occur that will prevent you completing it. If that is the case, this provides you with the opportunity to learn useful information for next time. Try to think about what happened. Could you have predicted the problem? What could you have done to prevent it? How could you put what you have learned into practice next time? Use the problem as an opportunity to learn.

Example

Someone who is facing symptoms might struggle to do the activities they usually did before. Even so, some life activities will still provide a sense of pleasure/achievement. For example, David may give a score of 6/10 for the pleasure he got from going for a walk in his garden, as before that he felt fed up and frustrated in the house. He may also rate it as 7/10 for achievement (he didn't want to go, and it felt difficult, but he managed it anyway).

This approach will allow you to plan in advance what you are going to do each day. The aim is to increase specific activity levels to boost your feelings of pleasure and sense of achievement.

> **KEY POINT**
> As we've already said before in this toolbox, we are not aiming to increase your total activity across the board. Instead the plan is to slowly increase *specific* activities that you have noticed give you a sense of pleasure or achievement. It may be that the thought of re-starting or increasing some of these activities seems daunting or impossible. The key is to use a step-by step plan where no step seems too large. Initially, using this approach may result in you doing less overall than you are at the moment, but then you will gradually increase the amount you do.

What does this say about any fears I had before or during the activity?

> **KEY POINT**
> no matter what happens – whether your plan is effective or seems to have failed badly – you can learn from it. Plan to take what you have learned into account in your next attempt.

Having planned and practised making this first change, the next key stage is for you to build upon this initial step so that you have a clear plan to move things forward still further.

SECTION 4: Planning the next steps

Now that you have considered how your planned activity went, the next step is to plan another activity to put into practice over the next week or so. This next step will build upon the initial step you have taken. Use what you have just learned about how your activity went to build on what you did.

You have the choice to:

- Repeat what you did.
- Take what you did and move it on one stage further.
- Select a new area of activity.

Planning to do an extra thing (even if it is a very small thing) each day that gives a sense of pleasure and/or achievement can be a useful approach.

Creating your own activity plan

As we said above, the next stage is to build upon this initial step so that you have a clear plan to move things forward. To do this, you need to think about your *short-*, *medium-* and *longer-term* targets. The key is to build one step upon another, so that each time you plan out and complete the seven-step approach you can then consider what the next step will be. Without this you may find that although you take some steps forward, these are all in different directions and you will lose your focus and motivation as a result.

Do:

- Plan to alter *only* one or two key activities over the next week.
- Produce an **activity plan** to slowly alter what you do in an effective and planned way.
- Ask yourself the **questions for effective change** to check that your activity is well planned.
- Write down your action plan in detail so that you will be able to put it into practice this week.
- Begin to *build in some other activities* that give you a sense of pleasure or achievement.

Don't:

- Choose something that is too ambitious a target.
- Try to alter too many activities all at once.

- Be very negative and think, 'Nothing can be done, what's the point, it's a waste of time.' Try to experiment to find out if this negative thinking is wholly accurate or helpful.

Use what you have learned earlier to write your activity plan. Plan what you will do and when you will do it. Learn from what happens so that you can keep putting what you have learned into practice. By doing this, you will be able to increase your activity levels in a planned, step-by-step way. By doing this, you will be slowly be able to re-build your confidence, and increase your feelings of pleasure and achievement.

Next steps: my activity plan

Day and date	**Planned activity** (Be specific. Is it a realistic plan? What do you have to do and when will you do it? What problems may occur? How can you overcome these problems?)	**Duration**	**Pleasure (P) (0–10)**	**Sense of achievement (A) (0–10)**
1				
2				
3				

As a general aim try to build in at least one thing each day that gives a sense of pleasure/achievement (P/A).

	Monday		Tuesday		Wednesday		Thursday		Friday		Saturday		Sunday	
	Activity	P/A	Activity	P/A	Activity	P/A	Activity	P/A	Activity	P/A	Activity	P/A	Activity	P/A
6 am														
7 am														
8 am														
9 am														
10 am														
11 am														
12 pm														
1 pm														
2 pm														
3 pm														
4 pm														
5 pm														
6 pm														
7 pm														
8 pm														
9 pm														
10 pm														

Diary record of the intensity of my main symptom/problem during the day. Date: ....

Time	*What am I doing at the moment?*	*Intensity of the main symptom (0–10)*
7am		
8am		
9am		
10am		
11am		
12pm		
1pm		
2pm		
3pm		
4pm		
5pm		
6pm		
7pm		
8pm		
9pm		
10pm		
11pm		

My current goal

What next step will you take? Make sure it is realistic and achievable.

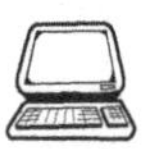

You can get additional help and support in problem solving at www.livinglifetothefull.com

Acknowledgements

The use of the Five Areas assessment model and associated language is used from the Overcoming Five Areas series by permission of Hodder Arnold Publishers and Dr C Williams. Illustrations are by Keith Chan and are reproduced with permission.

My Notes

Toolbox B

Practical problem solving

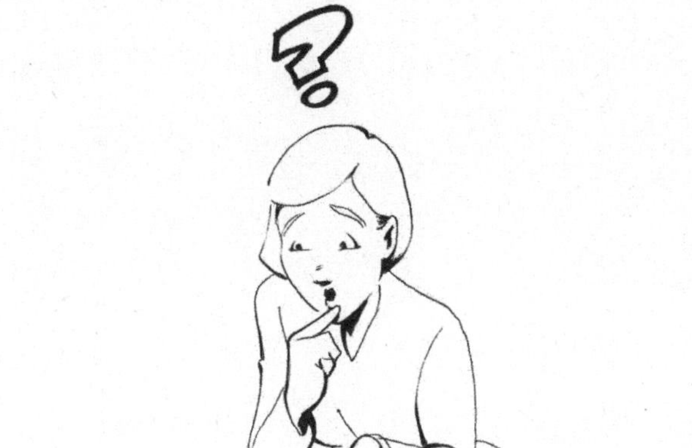

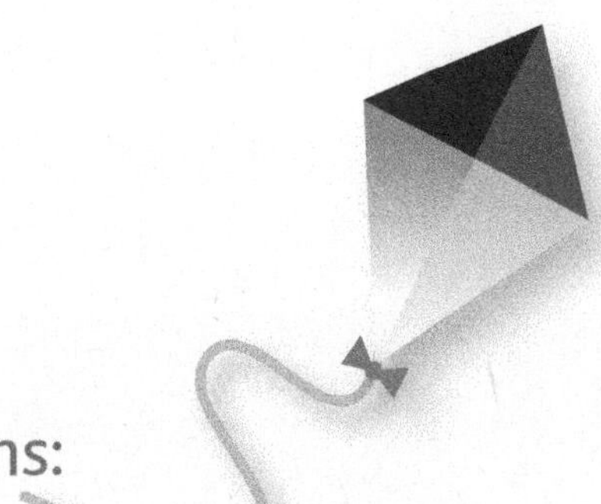

overcoming

functional neurological symptoms:
A Five Areas Approach

SECTION 1: Introduction

Everyone faces problems from time to time in their lives, and sometimes many problems are faced all at once. Problems are a normal part of daily life. No matter how hopeless you feel right now, in the past you will have faced problems that you have solved.

Task

Make a list of things that you have done well in the past. This will remind your of things you have coped with before and help you see your problem from a different perspective.

The reason for not managing to cope with problems is usually because too much has happened at the wrong time. When difficulties occur one at a time, it is usually easier to solve them. But when they happen one after the other, or all at once, it may seem much harder.

This may be particularly at times when people are experiencing symptoms. Health problems can reduce your ability to respond well to other problems in life. Opening letters, paying bills or keeping up with the house may just not seem as important when you are in pain, feel ill or have difficulties coping. These everyday difficulties are just one more source of unwanted pressure. Symptoms often seem worse when several life pressures occur up at the same time. These practical problems and life difficulties may include:

- Debts, housing or other difficulties.
- Problems in relationships with family, friends or colleagues, etc. Illness itself can sometimes affect relationships – and those around you may not know how best to help.
- Other difficult situations that you face such as problems at home or work (or lack of work, for example unemployment or problems with benefits).

When someone is finding that everything is 'too much' a common response is to 'do nothing'. In fact, people never do just nothing. They may not take any practical steps to overcome their problems, but you can be sure they are worrying about the problem but are doing this in a way that does not help sort it out.

A different approach is to tackle the problem in a planned, step-by-step manner. The principles of problem solving include:

- Defining the problem clearly.
- Approaching each problem separately *in turn*.
- Breaking down each problem into *smaller parts* that are then easier to solve.

This is the same approach as you have already learned to tackle reduced activity, avoidance or unhelpful behaviour. This part of the Toolbox will provide you with an opportunity to identify whether you have practical problems of your own. To help you with this, we will look at an example of how the seven-step approach we recommend can be applied with Paul and his money worries.

Below is a summary of several common situation, relationship and practical problems. Are any of these relevant to you?

Situation, relationship and practical problems

I have relationship difficulties (such as arguments)	Not relevant ☐	Yes ☐	No ☐
I can't really talk and receive support from my partner	Not relevant ☐	Yes ☐	No ☐
There is no one around who I can really talk to	Not relevant ☐	Yes ☐	No ☐
My children won't do what I tell them	Not relevant ☐	Yes ☐	No ☐
I have difficulties with money problems or debts	Not relevant ☐	Yes ☐	No ☐
I have difficulties with benefits	Not relevant ☐	Yes ☐	No ☐
There are problems with my flat/house	Not relevant ☐	Yes ☐	No ☐
I am having problems with my neighbours	Not relevant ☐	Yes ☐	No ☐
I don't have a job	Not relevant ☐	Yes ☐	No ☐
I have difficulties with colleagues at work	Not relevant ☐	Yes ☐	No ☐
Write down any other difficult situation, relationship and practical problems you may be facing. Remember these are external problems, so don't include 'internal' things like thoughts, emotions or your behaviours:			

SECTION 2: The seven steps to problem solving

In this approach, there are seven steps to problem solving. By working through the seven steps you can enable yourself to overcome your own problems. The first key step is to choose the problem you are going to tackle first.

Choosing a clear target

The key is to move from more general problem areas to a clearer target problem. So, for example, if you have a problem area such as 'I don't have enough money', a clearer target problem could be decided upon by asking yourself 'In what way does not having enough money cause me problems at the moment'. For example, it might cause problems because a credit card payment is due at the end of the month, and you don't have enough money to pay it.

One way of thinking about this process is to think of it as a **funnelling process**. You funnel down from the general problem area to a more specific target that you tackle first.

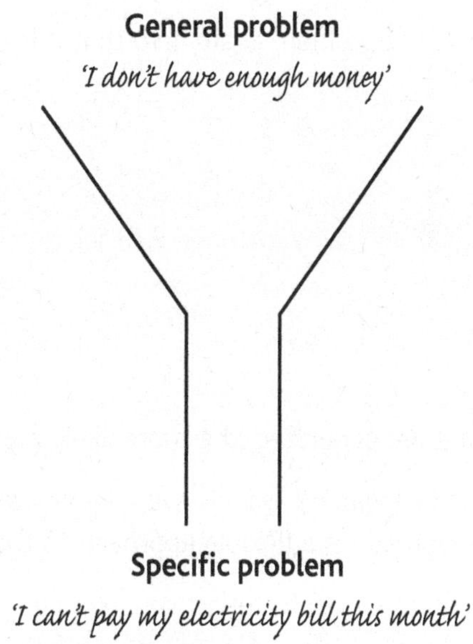

The funnel process: defining a specific problem.

A similar process can be used to help make any problem area clearer. For example, if the problem is 'I'm stressed by the behaviour of my neighbours', you might find it easier to be precise about the problem by asking yourself, 'Exactly what is it about my neighbours that is so stressful?' The same approach can therefore be used for tackling any practical problems you face – whether caused by illness or by other things in life.

Step 1: Identify and clearly define the problem as precisely as possible

Use the funnelling process to start with a general problem area. Work towards identifying a clearer target by again asking 'Exactly what is it about this problem area that is difficult for me at the moment?'

Try to clearly define your own problem as precisely as possible. Write it down and then ask yourself if this is a clear and focused problem.

My problem: (write down below)

Is this a clear, focused problem?

Yes ☐ No ☐

If you answered 'No', write the problem again it so that it is clear and focused.

Step 2: Think up as many solutions as possible to solve this initial problem

- The more solutions that are generated, the more likely a good one will emerge.
- Ridiculous ideas should be included as well, even if you would never choose them in practice. This can help you adopt a flexible approach to the problem.

Write a list of possible options. Useful questions to help you to think up possible solutions include:

- What *ridiculous* solutions can I include as well as more sensible ones?
- What helpful ideas would others (e.g. family, friends or colleagues at work) suggest?
- What approaches have I tried in the past in similar circumstances?
- What advice would I give a friend who was trying to tackle the same problem?

Example

Paul has debt problems because he has been on sick leave from work for several months and again cannot repay his credit card bill at the end of the month. He has a young baby and this adds to his stress. By focusing only on the money problem, he thinks up some possible options (including ridiculous ideas at first). Some of Paul's ideas are:

★ *Ignore the problem completely – it may go away.*

★ *Mug someone or rob a bank.*

★ *Try to arrange an overdraft from the bank and use this to pay off the bill.*

★ *Pay off a very small part of the money (the minimum asked for).*

★ *Switch my credit card payments to another credit card (one with a lower interest rate).*

★ *Speak to a counsellor with skills in debt repayments, such as the Citizens' Advice Bureau.*

★ *Speak to the credit card company to see if they will agree different repayment terms.*

Now brainstorm your own problem

Write in as many solutions as possible to your own problem. Include ridiculous ideas as well!

Step 3: Look at the advantages and disadvantages of each of the possible solutions

Think about the advantages and disadvantages of each possible solution. This will help you to decide which of the options are likely to be most practical and achievable for you.

Example: Paul weighs up the pros and cons of his solutions

The following is an extract from Paul's thoughts as he weighs up the pros and cons of each solution toward his target problem of finding a way to pay his credit card bill this month.

Suggestion	Advantages	Disadvantages
Ignore the problem completely	Easier in the short term with no embarrassment	The problems will worsen in the long term. It will have to be tackled some time
Mug someone or rob a bank	It would get me some money	It's unethical and wrong. I couldn't do it. I might be arrested. I couldn't harm someone else in this way. That's just ridiculous
Try to arrange a loan or overdraft with my bank	It would allow me a better rate of interest than paying off the high rate on my credit card. I could also spread the payments over a longer time. I have a good banking record and have been with them a number of years	How would I do this? It would be scary seeing the bank manager. They may also say no, even though I've been with them a number of years. They are a business after all
Pay off the minimum amount possible	Good short-term answer. It would prevent me defaulting the payments	The debt wouldn't get any smaller, and the interest rates will make it larger and larger. I'll never be able to pay it off
Switch to a cheaper credit card	This would be a lot cheaper. There are lots of good deals around with cheaper introductory rates	I would need to look at the small print of the different agreements and complete all the paperwork
Speak to a debt counsellor	I hear they can be very good	I'd feel embarrassed talking to them. How do you contact them?

Suggestion	Advantages	Disadvantages
Inform the credit card company and ask if they will agree different repayment terms	It would provide the company with clear information. It's in their best interests for me to keep up the payments. They may be flexible and allow a repayment break at a lower interest rate	It seems quite scary to do this

Now for your plan:

Think through the pluses and minuses of all the suggestions you came up within step 2. Write them below or on a separate piece of paper.

My suggestion	Advantages	Disadvantages

Step 4: Choose one of the solutions

In Paul's example, he decides to try to arrange a bank loan or overdraft. If his banking record had been worse, then choosing a different solution would have been sensible; however, this seems like a reasonable choice in his circumstances.

Your solution should be an option that is helpful and achievable. Use your answers from the last step to help decide the option that seems best for you.

This solution should be an option that fulfils the following two criteria:

Is it helpful?

Yes ☐ No ☐

Is it achievable?

Yes ☐ No ☐

My choice:

Step 5: Plan the steps needed to carry it out and apply the questions for effective change

This stage is a key part in the problem-solving process. The example below shows how Paul plans step 5.

Example: Paul plans his step 5

Paul has decided to arrange a bank loan or overdraft as it appears to be a reasonable solution. Other suggestions might also have worked, but this suggestion seems to be the most helpful and achievable based on his previous good banking record. Read Paul's answers to step 5:

I could phone my bank. I have the phone number on my bank statement. I'm quite nervous so I'm going to plan out what I am going to say in advance. I will phone up and ask to arrange a time to come in. I will tell them I'm having problems repaying my credit card because I'm off work sick. I'll ask if I can come in to see someone in the afternoon because I often feel better then. I think it's best if I also phone them in the afternoon. I'm more likely to get straight through to them then, and also I generally feel more confident after lunch.

Next, Paul needs to apply the **questions for effective change** to his plan to check how practical and achievable it is.

Is the planned solution one that:

★ Will be **useful** for understanding or changing how I am?

Yes ✓ No ☐

★ Is a **specific task** so that I will know when I have done it?

Yes ✓ No ☐

★ Is **realistic**: is it practical and achievable?

Yes ✓ No ☐

★ Makes clear **what** I'm going to do and **when** I'm going to do it?

Yes ✓ No ☐

★ Is an activity that won't be easily blocked or prevented by practical problems?

Yes ✓ No ☐

Now for your plan:

Write down (overleaf) the practical steps needed to carry out your own plan. Be as precise as possible. Think through *what* you are going to do, and *when* you are going to do it. Try to predict possible problems and work out how to avoid or deal with them.

When you have done this, apply the questions for effective change to your plan to check how practical and achievable your plan is:

Is my planned task one that:

- Will be useful for understanding or changing how I am?

Yes ☐ No ☐

- Is a specific task so that I will know when I have done it?

Yes ☐ No ☐

- Is realistic: is it practical and achievable?

Yes ☐ No ☐

- Makes clear *what* I am going to do and *when* I am going to do it?

Yes ☐ No ☐

- Is an activity that *won't be easily blocked* or prevented by practical problems?

Yes ☐ No ☐

If you have replied 'No' to any of these questions, revise your plan to try and overcome this. If it is difficult to do this, it may be that another solution from step 2 might be a better choice.

Step 6: Carry out the plan

Write down exactly what happened when you carried out your plan. As part of this summary, record what happened as you completed the plan, and also about what thoughts and feelings you experienced before, during and after your carried out the plan.

Step 7: Review the outcome

Example: What happened to Paul?

Paul phones the bank that afternoon as planned. Just before he does this, he feels quite scared. He predicts that the bank will humiliate him and turn his request down. Paul decides to try to challenge these fears by acting against them and phones the bank. At first the line is engaged. He tries again two minutes later and the phone is answered by an electronic answering service that asks him to make a selection of which service he wants from five options. Paul is surprised by this and becomes flustered and immediately puts the phone down.

His immediate thought is 'What an idiot – I should be able to do this'. Over the next few minutes, he is able to challenge this thought. He then decides to learn from what happened and try again. He therefore phones the bank again, but plans to have a pen and paper available to write down the different options. He finds that there is an option for those with payment difficulties. He selects this and arranges an appointment. When Paul goes to the bank he feels quite anxious and scared. He predicts that the manager will humiliate him and turn his request down, and that the credit card company will then demand immediate payment and issue a court summons.

Paul is surprised to be met by a friendly bank assistant rather than the manager. She says that she is Paul's personal account manager. She offers him a cup of tea, and they talk in a separate office so that their discussion is confidential. She tells him that this is a common problem. Because he has banked with them for several years and has a good banking record, she says there will be no problem in offering him a loan at a preferential rate. Paul agrees, and is happy with how things went. His fears were not correct. He was offered a loan. This is at a rate that he can afford.

Paul's review:

In this case, Paul's plan went smoothly. This shows he had planned it well, and had been realistic about his chances of a loan.

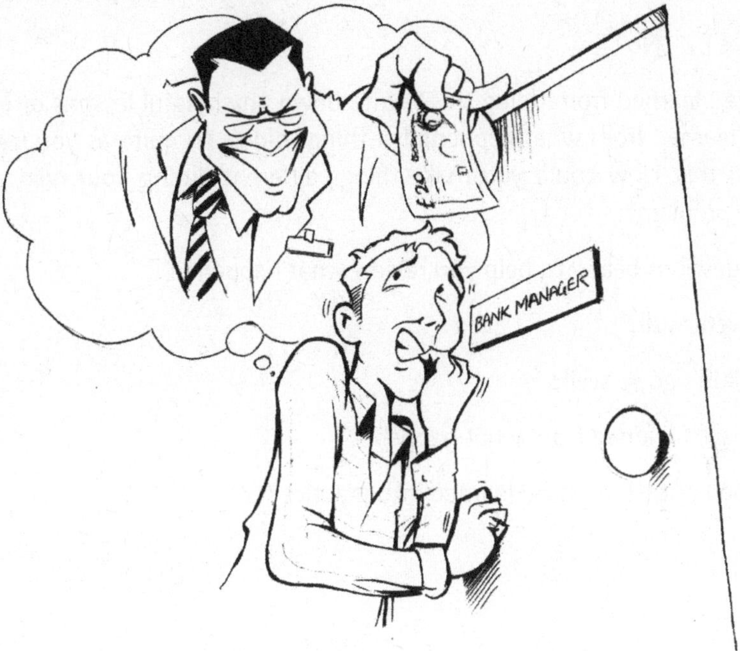

What if Paul had been turned down?

Even if he had been turned down, there are lots of useful things he could have learned from the process:

- ★ That there is usually more than one solution – he has other possible solutions left that he can try.
- ★ His fears are not always accurate. Although he didn't get the loan his very worst fears weren't correct. He wasn't humiliated. He didn't even see a nasty bank manager. At least he got a free cup of tea out of the bank.
- ★ He has practised the seven-step plan and can learn from it and put what he has learned into practice next time.

Now for your plan: What happened when you carried out your plan?
Complete the checklist and answer the questions that follow:

Was the selected approach successful?

Yes ☐ No ☐

Did it help deal with the target problem?

Yes ☐ No ☐

Were there any disadvantages to using this approach?

Yes ☐ No ☐

What have I learned from doing this? Write down any helpful lessons or information you have learned from what happened. If things didn't go quite as you hoped, try to learn from this. How could you make things different during your next attempt to tackle the problem?

Use the questions below to help you review what happened.

- What went well?
- What didn't go so well?
- What have I learned from what happened?
- How can I put what I have learned into practice?

Even if things haven't gone well you can learn from this and take it into account with your next plan. Also, even if some things haven't turned out right in the approach, much will have gone well.

Whatever the practical problem, the same approach can be used. You can apply it both to practical problems that have arisen because of your symptoms, or to problems that have any other cause.

Planning the next steps

You have now practised this approach for the first time. The next step is to build slowly on what you have done in a step-by-step way. You have the choice to:

- Stop using the approach if you have overcome all your problems.
- Work on other aspects of the same problem.
- Select a new problem area to tackle.

You must decide for yourself which decision is the best for you.

KEY POINT

Remember, it is not possible to deal with every problem all at once. In fact, if you try to change everything at once you will be potentially setting yourself up to fail. Instead, by focusing on one clear target problem at a time, you can use the same seven-step plan to tackle any future problems.

SECTION 3: Conclusion

Problem solving is a technique that needs to be practised. You will improve your skills in this approach by using them. Try to learn from anything that goes wrong and keep practising so that using this approach becomes second nature whenever you face a problem.

Putting what you have learned into practice

- Choose one or two problems only and use the seven-step problem-solving approach now and during the next two or three weeks.
- Write down all the steps as you do them, and review for yourself the progress you make. If you have difficulties, just do what you can.
- If you have found any aspects of this workbook unhelpful, upsetting or confusing, try to discuss this with your healthcare practitioner or someone else whose opinion you trust.

My current goal

Write down your next goal. Make sure it is realistic and achieveable.

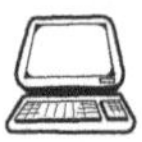

You can get additional help and support in problem solving at www.livinglifetothefull.com

Acknowledgements

The use of the Five Areas assessment model and associated language is used from the Overcoming Five Areas series by permission of Hodder Arnold Publishers and Dr C Williams. Illustrations are by Keith Chan and are reproduced by permission.

My Notes

Toolbox C

How to become more assertive

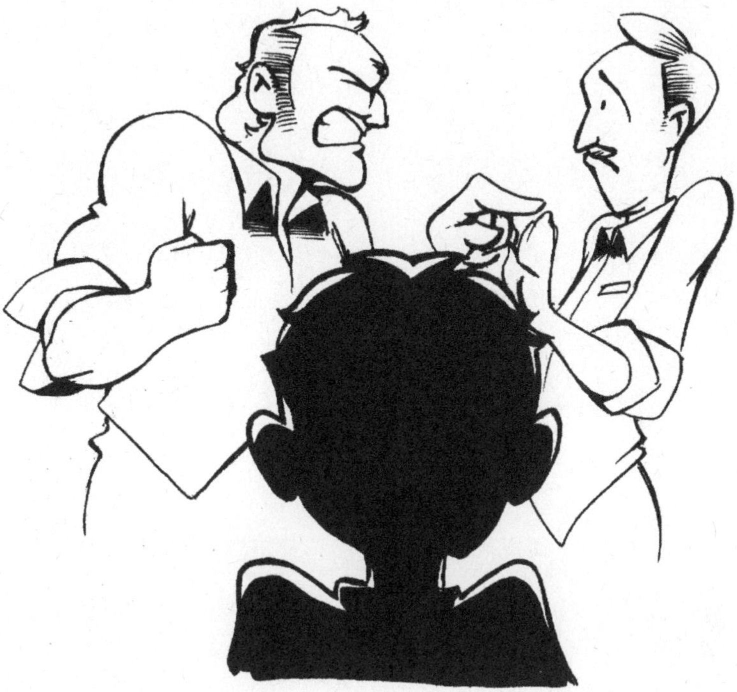

overcoming

functional neurological symptoms:
A Five Areas Approach

SECTION 1: Introduction

At some times in life, however confident a person is, it can be hard to deal with certain difficult situations. Examples of these could be:

- Communicating feelings to partners, family or friends.
- Expressing yourself to your healthcare practitioner or hospital doctor.
- Dealing with unhelpful shop assistants, or with poor service in a restaurant or garage.
- Dealing with angry or difficult colleagues at work.

Sometimes people deal with these situations by losing their temper, by saying nothing or by giving in. This may leave them feeling unhappy, angry, out of control and may not actually solve the problem. When you are physically unwell and feel tired, ground down or in pain this can become an area of even greater difficulty. When people have become unwell, they often change their ways of relating to people and sometimes allow others to make decisions for them and tell them what's best.

What is assertiveness?

Assertiveness is being able to stand up for yourself, making sure your feelings are considered and not letting other people treat you like a doormat. It is not the same as aggressiveness. You can be assertive without being forceful or rude. It is stating clearly what you expect and insisting that your rights are considered. Assertion is a skill that can be *learnt*. It is a way of communicating and behaving with others that helps people to become more confident and aware of their needs and themselves.

Where does assertiveness come from?

As we grow up we model ourselves upon those around us, for example our parents, teachers and friends, and other influences such as television and the magazines we read. This may teach us to react *passively*, *aggressively* or *assertively*. We may have seen people we love act in a particular way when they are unwell and adopt these patterns ourselves.

What are aggressive, passive and assertive behaviours?

Aggression is the opposite of assertion. Aggression is expressing your own feelings, needs, rights and opinions in a demanding and angry way. There is *no respect* for other people's feelings, needs, rights and opinions. Your own needs are seen as being more important than other people's. Their needs are ignored or dismissed. It means focusing on your own rights, but doing so in such a way that you violate the rights of other people. The aim of aggression is to win, if necessary at the expense of others. An example of this might be when you have planned something for a person to do and they do not feel physically well enough or able to take part, but rather than expressing how they feel, they become angry with you for having planned the activity in the first place. However, when adjusting to your symptoms it is normal to feel angry and frustrated as you and also those around you adjust to how you are. How you express your anger and frustration is the key to managing your relationships with others.

Task

Try to think of a time when someone else has been aggressive with you and ignored your opinion. How did it make you feel about them and yourself?

In the *short term*, the aggressive person often feels more powerful, however, in the longer term it can cause resentment in others.

Passive behaviour is *not* expressing your feelings, needs, rights and opinions. Instead you see other people's needs as *more* important than your own. You may be frightened to say what you think in case your beliefs are ridiculed. The aim of passive behaviour is to **avoid conflict** at all times and to **please others**. Everyone else is seen as better or more deserving than you. It involves bottling up your own feelings or expressing them in indirect or unhelpful ways. The effect of passive behaviour is loss of self-esteem, stress, anger and depression.

Passive behaviour may cause others to become increasingly irritated with you and to develop a lack of respect for you. This may lead to a pattern where others expect you to give in and do not take your opinion into account. An example of this might be if we allow someone to tell us we're not able to do something when actually we would like to try. Instead of expressing our own view we allow the other person to decide what's best for us.

The good news is that if you have noticed that you tend to respond in aggressive or passive ways, you can learn new ways of communicating. In contrast to aggression and passivity there is a third way to respond – the assertive way.

SECTION 2: Elements of assertion

Assertion is expressing your own feelings, needs, rights and opinions with a respect for other people's feelings, needs, rights and opinions. Assertion is not about winning. It is concerned with being able to walk away feeling that you put across what you wanted to say.

- **Feelings**: In assertion, you are able to express your feelings in a direct and honest way.
- **Needs**: You have needs that have to be met otherwise you feel undervalued, anxious, angry or sad.
- **Rights**: You have basic human rights and it is possible to stand up for your own rights in such a way that you do not violate another person's rights.
- **Opinions**: You have something to contribute irrespective of other people's views.

Task

Try to think about a time when someone else has been assertive with you and respected your opinion. How did you feel about them and yourself?

About me – I felt: (write here):

About them – I felt: (write here):

In assertiveness you ask for what you want directly, openly and honestly. You respect your own opinions and rights. You expect others to do the same. You do not:

- Violate people's rights.
- Expect other people to magically know what you want.
- Freeze with anxiety and avoid difficult issues.

The result is improved self-confidence and mutual respect from others.

The rules of assertion

I have the right to:

1. Respect myself – who I am and what I do.

2. Recognise my own needs as an individual – that is separate from what is expected of me in particular roles, such as 'wife', 'husband', 'partner', 'son', 'daughter'.

3. Make clear 'I' statements about how I feel and what I think. For example, 'I feel very uncomfortable with your decision.'

4. Allow myself to make mistakes. Recognising that it is normal to make mistakes.

5. Change my mind, if I choose.

6. Ask for 'thinking it over time'. For example, when people ask you to do something, you have the right to say, 'I would like to think it over and I will let you know by the end of the week.'

7. Allow myself to enjoy my successes, that is by being pleased with what I have done and sharing it with others.

8. Ask for what I want, rather than hoping someone will notice what I want.

9. Recognise that I am not responsible for the behaviour of other adults.

10. Respect other people and their right to be assertive and expect the same in return.

Task

Think about how much you believe each of these rules. How much do you put them into practice in your own life at the moment?

I have the right to:	*Do I believe this rule is true?*	*Have I applied this in the last week?*
1. Respect myself	Yes ☐ No ☐	Yes ☐ No ☐
2. Recognise my own needs as an individual independent of others	Yes ☐ No ☐	Yes ☐ No ☐
3. Make clear 'I' statements about how I feel and what I think. For example, 'I feel very uncomfortable with your decision'	Yes ☐ No ☐	Yes ☐ No ☐
4. Allow myself to make mistakes	Yes ☐ No ☐	Yes ☐ No ☐
5. Change my mind	Yes ☐ No ☐	Yes ☐ No ☐
6. Ask for 'thinking it over time'	Yes ☐ No ☐	Yes ☐ No ☐
7. Allow myself to enjoy my successes	Yes ☐ No ☐	Yes ☐ No ☐
8. Ask for what I want, rather than hoping someone will notice what I want	Yes ☐ No ☐	Yes ☐ No ☐
9. Recognise that I am not responsible for the behaviour of other adults	Yes ☐ No ☐	Yes ☐ No ☐
10. Respect other people and their right to be assertive and expect the same in return	Yes ☐ No ☐	Yes ☐ No ☐

SECTION 3: Assertiveness techniques

It is possible to put these rights into practice by practising a number of assertiveness techniques.

How to use assertiveness techniques

'Broken record'

This is a useful technique and can work in virtually any situation. You plan what it is you want to say by repeating over and over again what it is you want or need. During the conversation keep returning to your prepared lines. State clearly and precisely exactly what it is you need or want. (e.g. 'I can't lend you any money ... I'm sorry, but I can't lend you any money ...'). Don't be put off by clever arguments or by what the other person says. Once you have prepared the lines you want to say, you can relax. **There is nothing that can defeat this tactic.**

This approach is useful in situations where your rights are being ignored and in saying 'no' to things.

Example: Using the 'broken record' technique

Joe: 'I think you should stay in bed today and not go for a walk.'

Caroline: 'I want to get up today and go for a short walk, it's part of my plan.'

Joe: 'You had a bad day yesterday and should stay in bed. You never listen to good advice.'

Caroline: 'I am getting up and going for a short walk.'

Joe: 'I'm only telling you what's best for you. The rest will do you good.'

Caroline: 'I know you feel your advice is for my benefit but I want to get up and go for that short walk; it's important I stick with my plan.'

Saying 'no'

Sometimes 'No' seems to be the hardest word to say. Sometimes you can be drawn into situations that you don't want to be in. You avoid saying this one simple word. The images you recall with saying 'no' sometimes prevent you from using 'no' when you need it. We may be scared of being seen as mean, difficult and selfish, or of being rejected by others.

Do I have problems saying 'No'?

Yes ☐ No ☐

If yes: Saying 'no' can be both important and helpful. Try to practise saying 'no' by using the following principles. Try to:

- Be straightforward but not rude so that you can make your point effectively.
- Tell the person if you are finding it difficult. Avoid apologising and giving elaborate reasons for saying 'no'. You are allowed to say no if you don't want to do things.
- Remember that it is better in the long run to be truthful than breed resentment and bitterness within you by giving in.

It may be that you have fears of how others may see you if you say no. Use the techniques in Workbook 5 to challenge thoughts such as these.

Scripting

Scripting involves planning out in advance in your mind, or on paper, exactly what you want to say. A good way to begin to practise scripting is to write down what you would say *before* you go into a situation. It uses a four-stage plan that covers events, feelings, needs and consequences.

- **Event**: Say what it is you are talking about. Let the other person know precisely what situation you are referring to.
- **Feelings**: Express how the event mentioned affects your own feelings. Opinions can be argued with, feelings cannot. Expressing your feelings clearly can prevent a lot of confusion.
- **Needs**: People are not mind readers. You need to tell them what you need. Otherwise people cannot fulfil your needs and this can lead to resentment and misunderstandings.
- **Consequences**: Tell the person that if they fulfil your need, there will be a positive consequence for both of you. Be specific about the consequences.

Example: Scripting

Kate: 'Hi, how are you?'

Nicola: 'Fine and you?'

Kate: 'Okay but I saw Sandra yesterday. She said she was sorry to hear that I wasn't well. She told me she'd read a magazine and thought she knew what was wrong with me. I told you about my symptoms in confidence. I didn't expect you to go round telling everyone.' **(Event)**

Nicola: 'I thought Sandra was good friends with you. I really didn't think you'd mind. She asked how you were. What was I supposed to say?'

Kate: 'Sandra's okay but she likes to gossip with everyone. I'm angry and upset that you've discussed me with her. I just feel let down. My symptoms are hard enough without other people telling me what they think is wrong.' **(Feeling)**

Nicola: 'I didn't think. I'm sorry.'

Kate: 'You're one of my best friends. I need to be able to talk to you about things in confidence without you telling everyone else about it.' **(Need)**

Nicola: 'I feel the same. I don't know what made me say anything to Sandra. Let's not spoil our friendship over this.'

Kate: 'Okay, but let's agree not to discuss each other's problems with anyone.' **(Consequence)**

Task

Identify an area where you could use scripting. Plan out what you want to say here:

Event:

Feeling:

Needs:

Consequence:

SECTION 4: Conclusion

Assertiveness is an attitude and a way of life. You can slowly learn to be more assertive, or to regain the assertive way you used to be, through practice. Remember that although change can seem difficult at first, it is possible.

Putting what you have learned into practice

Write down and **pin up** the rules for assertion in visible places about the house (e.g. on the fridge door and by your bed, etc.). Try to put into practice what you have learned. Experiment using the broken record and scripting approaches. Begin to say 'no' – politely and assertively. Don't expect to change everything immediately, however, with practice you can gain confidence in your ability to be assertive. If you have difficulties just do what you can.

My current goal

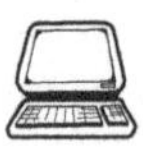

You can get additional help and support in problem solving at www.livinglifetothefull.com

Acknowledgements

The use of the Five Areas assessment model and associated language is used from the Overcoming Five Areas series by permission of Hodder Arnold Publishers and Dr C Williams. Illustrations are by Keith Chan and are reproduced by permission.

My notes

Toolbox D

Healthy living

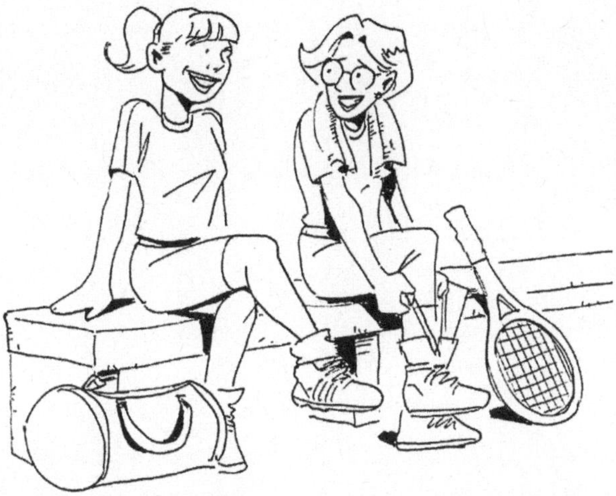

overcoming
functional neurological symptoms:
A Five Areas Approach

SECTION 1: Why consider healthy living?

This workbook provides a summary of general information about healthy living. Considering issues such as diet and balanced living can be important aspects of self-care. You will learn about:

- Relaxation and effective breathing techniques.
- Smoking and alcohol and their impact on people's lives.
- A balanced diet and healthy eating.
- The impact of caffeine in coffee and other drinks.
- How to improve sleep and establish a regular sleep/wake pattern.
- How to put what you've learned into practice in how you feel and what you do.

A person's general physical well-being has an effect on how they feel, regardless of the specific symptoms they are experiencing. The better care you can take of your body, the more you can expect to benefit.

> **KEY POINT**
> **Healthy living can have a positive impact on how you feel, despite your symptoms.**

SECTION 2: Learning to relax and how to change your breathing

Relaxation techniques

There are many methods of relaxation. If you have something that works for you, do use it. Some people relax by gardening, walking, swimming, reading a book or almost any activity. However, your symptoms might mean that you have stopped participating in activities that you previously found relaxing.

Relaxation is also a skill that can be learned and becomes easier and easier with practice. Initially it is advisable to practise relaxation at least once per day for up to 30 minutes. It can also be helpful to plan times for relaxation into your day. For example, plan to use the relaxation approach at certain times, such as unwinding just before bed, or at times you feel stressed, anxious or angry.

If you decide to complete an activity schedule to help plan your day, such as the one given on page 198, a period of relaxation can be included in that. Even if you don't believe that relaxation can be of benefit to you, try one of the techniques for a week as an experiment.

KEY POINT

Initially when you try to practise relaxation it is important that you let people know that you need some quiet time. Unplug the phone, close the curtains, make sure you're comfortable; if you will be putting on music, ensure it has no lyrics or memories associated with it or your mind may wander. Once you have become more practised in this technique, you should be able to call on these skills in any place and at any time to combat stress.

Free online relaxation resources: A number of free web-based relaxation resources are available free of charge at www.livinglifetothefull.com

Diaphragmatic breathing

You may find this of benefit if overbreathing is a problem for you. You can find out if this is the case in Workbook 2 in the section on hyperventilation. The following exercise will help you to regulate the body's need for oxygen and re-establish a regular breathing pattern.

- Sit in a chair, relax your whole body and ensure the chair supports your lower back.

- Ensure both your feet are placed grounded on the floor.
- Put one hand over your stomach and the other at the top of your chest.
- Breathe in gently and imagine you are filling the lower part of your stomach with air.
- The hand that is over your stomach will rise and the hand that is on your chest should stay relatively still. Keep breathing slowly and deeply.
- When you breathe out the hand over your stomach should sink slightly.
- Repeat again, it can be helpful to imagine in your mind's eye that you are filling a balloon with air and as you breathe out this is deflating.
- Your breathing should remain slow and rhythmic, and if your mind wanders bring yourself back to the here and now, and focus on your breathing. This should be continued for at least 10 minutes.

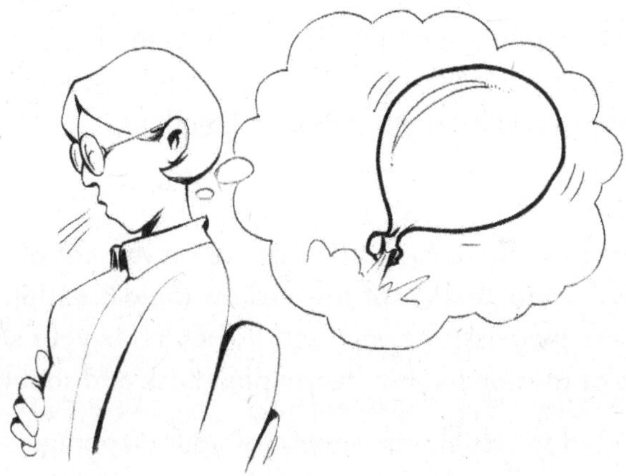

Hints and tips to re-establish a diaphragmatic breathing pattern

The following exercises will help you to establish a relaxed diaphragmatic breathing pattern. By practising, you will be able to breathe like this throughout the rest of the day without even having to think about it. Try to persevere. It will take about a week or more to notice a significant change. If you have chest problems such as emphysema, heart disease or chronic obstructive airways disease, discuss the exercises with your doctor before using them.

1 Breathe in through your nose while counting silently to three.

Then:

2 Record the length of time you can breathe out while saying:

s ————————→ (i.e. sssssssssssssssssss).

Do this once or twice as a baseline to allow comparison later as you practise the other exercises. Concentrate on slowly controlling how you breathe out using your diaphragm. You will feel this muscle working as you do this. Aim to slowly increase the time you take as you breathe out. An average would be 12–15 seconds with no discomfort and no excessive tension.

3 Breathe out slowly as a sigh:

hhh ——————→

Again, feel your diaphragm gently tense as you breathe out.

4 Breathe in gently through your nose over a silent, slow count of three.

5 Then pause for a count of three.

6 Finally breathe out slowly through your mouth for a count of three. Take only one or two breaths and relax. Settle your breathing before trying again to avoid any dizziness.

As you practise this, gently extend the time spent breathing out to a count of three, four and so on. Try to reach eight to 10. Do this in a relaxed way that isn't rushed. The aim is to re-establish a relaxed rhythm to your breathing.

HELPFUL HINTS

Be aware of any tension or excessive movement of your shoulders. This is a useful marker of the shallow rapid breathing that is a problem in anxiety. As you breathe out, relax your shoulders and be aware of tension in your neck, upper back and shoulders.

Do: watch for visible movement of your diaphragm. Remember, the diaphragm is situated just below your ribs at the top of your stomach.

Don't: move your shoulders. You want to reduce any anxious over-breathing and tension in the upper part of your chest.

7 Breathe in gently, then breathe out slowly through your mouth. Again, correct any shoulder movement and reduce any anxious overbreathing with the upper part of your chest.

8 Produce the following sounds. By doing so you are controlling the rate of air being breathed out by using the diaphragm. Try each exercise on three occasions but don't necessarily do all the exercises in one sitting. These exercises teach you how to create gentle variations in volume controlled by the diaphragm.

Ssssssss

ssssssss

sssssSSSSSsssss

sssssSSSSSssssssSSSSSsssss

shshshshsh

shshshshsh

sh------sh------sh

sh------sh------sh------sh------sh------sh------sh

By practising each of the exercises several times a day, you should notice that your breathing develops a more natural and relaxed rhythm over several weeks.

Fast relaxation for mental tension

Find a comfortable sitting position. Close your eyes and think of a relaxing place you have been before that you felt was ideal for physical and mental relaxation. It should be a quiet environment, maybe by the sea or a river or even in your own garden. If you cannot think of an actual place then create one in your mind.

Now imagine yourself in that relaxing place. Imagine you are seeing the colours, hearing the sounds, feeling the temperature or breeze. Sit back and enjoy the sense of relaxation. Feel the peace and calm and imagine your whole mind being renewed and refreshed.

After five or 10 minutes open your eyes and stretch. Be aware that you can return to this place in your mind whenever you desire, and can achieve peace and tranquillity there.

Fast relaxation for mind and body

If you become aware of increasing stress or tension (e.g. clenched jaw or gritted teeth) or just generally feeling uptight then stop and become aware of how you are feeling. The following can be useful when you are around other people as they will not be aware of what you are doing – however, you will need to be able to sit down, or miss out the exercise involving your legs.

- Take a small breath and hold it for approximately seven seconds.
- At the same time, tense your leg muscles by crossing your legs at the ankles, pressing down with the upper leg whilst trying to lift the lower leg.

- Slowly breathe out, saying the word 'relax' to yourself while letting all the tension go from your muscles.
- Take a small breath and hold for seven seconds.
- With your hands in your lap press palm against palm, pushing down with the top hand while trying to lift the bottom.
- Slowly breathe out, saying the word 'relax' to yourself while letting all the tension go from your muscles.
- Repeat these exercises until you feel relaxed.

Some difficulties with relaxation exercises

Some people find it difficult to relax even when using some of the techniques described. The two main reasons are a lack of practice and the presence of unhelpful thinking that interferes with the relaxation process.

'I don't like how relaxation makes me feel'

Sometimes people experience emotions as a result of relaxation that can feel distressing. This is often because they have been trying hard to 'keep a lid' on these emotions and the combined physical, emotional and mental effects of relaxation result in a letting go of emotions as well as a letting go of tension.

This should actually be viewed as relaxation 'working'. Through practice, you will increase your knowledge and confidence of how you experience these emotions in your mind and body.

'I'm just too wound up to relax'

Relaxation may take longer when you are very tense. Experiment with combinations of all the techniques described, perhaps starting with the muscular relaxation described below.

Muscular relaxation

Once you have regulated your breathing and feel comfortable with those techniques you can move on to the rest of the body.

1. Start with the toes. Curl them round and press your feet down, tensing up as you breath IN and holding for several seconds. Then relax the muscles as you breathe OUT.
2. Move up the leg to the calf muscles. Tense them as you breathe IN and hold for several seconds and then relax them as you breathe OUT.

Use this approach to work up through your body, tensing your thigh muscles, your buttocks, your stomach, arms, shoulders, jaw and face muscles. Then bring yourself back to focus on your breathing. This should be continued for at least 10 minutes.

KEY POINT

Relaxation can sometimes be difficult to achieve. We live in a world that can make many demands of us. Taking time – your time – to relax is an important commitment. Tackling tension involves both learning relaxation skills but also learning to tackle problems, and challenge worrying thoughts. All three approaches can be used together.

SECTION 3: Tips for a healthy lifestyle

Smoking

The best advice about smoking is that if you do smoke you should stop – or at least cut down if you can. Even reducing how much you smoke can be helpful, as evidence shows that the more you smoke, the more your health is at risk.

If you find yourself unable to stop completely, try to cut down to fewer than five cigarettes a day and leave long portions of the day without a cigarette. You may find it helpful to discuss the use of other approaches (such as nicotine patches) with your doctor.

Most health centres and doctors' surgeries have smoking cessation clinics or groups that can also help.

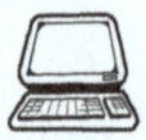

There are various websites and telephone support lines providing helpful advice and support, e.g. www.givingupsmoking.co.uk. Do an internet search or use a telephone directory to identify your local smoking advisory service. A linked little book (*Stop smoking in five minutes*) is available from www.fiveareas.com.

Diet and healthy eating

Symptoms can cause a variety of difficulties related to eating. You can sometimes experience a marked reduction in your appetite and only want to pick at food and experience little or no pleasure from it. Sometimes there is a marked increase in appetite as a side effect of medication. Also many people use food as a comfort or as a substitute for things they no longer do. The result can be weight gain or loss.

There are no 'special diets' to be recommended for people with functional neurological symptoms, but most experts agree that eating a healthy balanced diet gives your body the best chance of recovery. In order to identify any areas in your diet that are out of balance it might be helpful to keep a **food diary** over a few 'typical' days. A blank diary for your use is given below. Each day you should record:

- What and how much you eat.
- At what time you eat it.
- Any factors, such as how you felt or any symptoms that affected your choice of food.

My food diary

Food eaten	*Day and time*	*Note any altered feelings or any symptoms affecting your choice of food*

What is a healthy balanced diet?

Research suggests that eating large amounts of sugar and refined foods such as white bread, sugary food, heat-up meals, etc. can sometimes increase irritability. If you have bowel difficulties as part of your symptoms, it will be a good idea to increase your fibre intake. How you can do this is described below. An additional advantage is that this also helps to stop rapid changes in blood sugar levels, which can affect your energy levels and prevent food cravings.

KEY POINT

Aim for a diet that is *low* in fat and sugar and *high* in fibre.

Try to eat three meals a day, and if you also usually snack, try healthy snacks such as fresh or dried fruit or nuts. These foods release energy slowly and prevent large changes in blood glucose, which can result in faintness and hunger.

Some small things that can make a difference

The following changes will help you eat more healthily.

- Eat one more piece of fruit per day. Try to aim for five portions of fruit or vegetables a day.
- Have oily fish (e.g. salmon, sardines, mackerel) at least once per week.
- Eat one fewer take-away meal per week.
- Read up on healthy eating so that you can make healthy eating choices.
- Reduce your overall sugar intake. For example, don't add sugar to hot drinks or cooking, eat fewer sweets and chocolate. Consider using low-calorie sugar substitutes.
- Increase your fibre intake. Swap every other white bread loaf you buy for a wholemeal one. Eat a breakfast rich in fibre such as wheat cereals, muesli or porridge. Increasing fibre in your diet should be done gradually.
- Reduce your salt intake. A key way to achieve this is to avoid too many processed meals, such as microwave meals, as these are often high in salt. Taste food before adding salt. Check for low salt or low sodium on packaging.

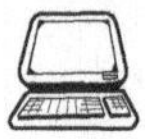

A linked little book that addresses healthy eating and how to achieve a healthy weight (*Live longer: have a heart attack*) is available from www.fiveareas.com.

Caffeine

Caffeine is a chemical that is present in coffee, tea, cocoa, fizzy drinks such as cola, and some painkillers. We often drink caffeine because it tends to make us feel more alert or energetic. However, caffeine constricts blood vessels, which can result in decreased blood flow and oxygen delivered to your muscles. This can increase pain and spasm. Caffeine also affects your ability to get off to sleep and can worsen the quality of sleep. Due to its stimulant effects caffeine can also cause an increase in blood pressure and heart rate. People can also build up a physical tolerance to caffeine. This is a technical term to mean that your body becomes used to it and you need to drink more and more to feel the same effect. So if you rely on caffeine as a pick me up, you can end up needing more and more to have the same effect. Withdrawal symptoms such as headaches, poor sleep, or feeling nervous or tense can occur if you abruptly stop drinking caffeine.

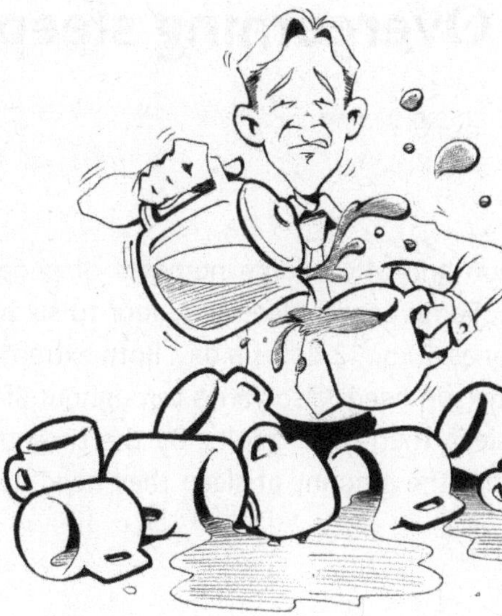

Because of this, any cuts in caffeine intake should occur slowly over a few days. When you are reducing your caffeine intake it is important to drink lots of fluids to keep you well hydrated.

> **KEY POINT**
> **It is important to limit the amount of caffeine you use, particularly if you experience fatigue.**

Further information

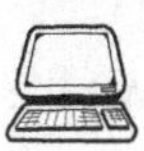

If this is an area of interest for you there are lots of helpful healthy eating resources, such as:

- Websites:
  - www.llttf.com
  - www.food.gov.uk
- Telephone helpline: 0845 278 8878.

A variety of books and leaflets will also be available in your local library. General, evidence-based information on healthy living is available at www.ebandolier.com.

SECTION 4: Overcoming sleep difficulties

What is sleep?

Sleep problems are common and affect large numbers of people. There is a wide normal healthy sleep range. Some people sleep only four to six hours a day whereas others can sleep for as many as 10 or 12 hours a day. Both extremes are quite normal. The amount of sleep each person needs also varies throughout life. Babies and young children need a lot more sleep than older adults. By the time they reach their 60s or 70s, many people find that the amount of sleep they need has dropped by up to several hours a night.

What is insomnia?

Insomnia is an *inability to sleep*. Many people have problems sleeping from time to time. Insomnia often starts after an upsetting life event or can be caused by a person's lifestyle. A number of different psychological problems can also upset sleep. They include anxiety, depression and stress at work or in relationships. For example, a person who experiences depression may find that it takes them several hours to get off to sleep. They then may wake up several hours earlier than normal feeling unrested or on edge. External factors such as noisy neighbours or having a young baby who needs to be fed during the night can leave a person lacking in sleep.

A Five Areas assessment of sleeplessness

The following factors can worsen sleep. Think about whether they affect your own life.

Area 1: Situation, relationship and practical problems (that is, people and events around you)

Physical environment

Is your bed comfortable? What about the temperature of the room where you sleep? If the room is either very cold or very hot this might make sleeping difficult. Is the room very noisy? Is there too much light to sleep? If bright lights such as streetlights come through your curtains, this can also prevent sleep.

Do I sleep in a poor sleep environment?

Yes ☐ No ☐

If you answered 'yes', the following are specific things that you can do.

- **Poor mattress.** If your mattress is old, try turning it over, rotating it or changing it. Try adding extra support such as a board underneath.
- **Too hot/cold.** If it is too hot open a window or use a fan. If it is too cold, think about insulation, secondary or double glazing, etc., or add an extra blanket or duvet.
- **Problems with noise.** Reduce noise if you can. Speak to noisy neighbours to ask them to turn down their television or music. Have you thought about fitting double-glazing or internal plastic sheeting over windows to reduce noise? You might also buy earplugs from a chemist to block the noise. However, if you have a baby, you may need to be able to hear them if he or she wakes up in the night so it may not be possible to stop all these noises. If you have a partner, sharing who gets up in turn in response to crying may help. So if you are expressing or bottle feeding and have access to a spare room, try to spend occasional nights sleeping in a different room with no child monitor to wake you up.
- **Problems with excessive light.** Consider changing your curtains. Add a thicker lining or blackout lining. If cost is a problem, a black plastic bin bag can be an effective blackout blind. Staple or stick it to the curtain rail.

Area 2: Symptoms

Symptoms can cause sleeplessness at times. Also if your body is used to using energy every day and you have now become inactive this can contribute to sleeplessness.

Are symptoms keeping me awake?

Yes ☐ No ☐

If you answered 'yes', and physical symptoms are keeping you awake, discuss this with your healthcare practitioner in case there is any additional help they can offer. Sometimes symptoms of depression or anxiety can worsen symptoms such as pain, in which case treating the low or anxious mood can help to reduce this.

Area 3: Thinking

Anxious thoughts are a common cause of sleeplessness. Anxious thoughts may be about worries in general. They can also sometimes focus on worry about not sleeping. You may worry that it will not be possible to sleep at all, or that sleeplessness will reduce your ability to be effective during the day/at work, etc. These unrealistic fears prevent you getting off to sleep. Other common fears include worries that your brain or body will be harmed by lack of sleep and that this may worsen the symptoms or how you cope with them.

In sleep, there is a reduction in tension levels leading your body and brain to begin to relax and drop off to sleep. In contrast, in anxiety the brain becomes overly alert.

You end up mulling things over again and again. This is the exact opposite of what is needed to get off to sleep. Worrying thoughts are therefore both a cause and effect of poor sleep.

Do I worry about things in general?

Yes ☐ No ☐

If you answered 'yes', read Workbook 5 (Noticing and changing unhelpful thinking).

Do I worry about not sleeping?

Yes ☐ No ☐

If you answered 'yes', jot down notes of your worries on a notepad. You will need to challenge any catastrophic fears about the consequences of not sleeping. Studies show that most people do not need very much sleep at all to be physically and mentally healthy. In sleep research laboratories, it has been found that many people who experience insomnia *actually sleep far more than they think*. Sometimes people who are in a light level of sleep *dream that they are awake*. You therefore may be sleeping more than you think. You also need to know that sleep deprivation does *not* have a catastrophic impact on your brain or body. It is possible to function effectively with very little sleep each night.

Task

If worrying thoughts are problems for you, read Workbook 5 (Noticing and changing unhelpful thinking).

Area 4: Behaviour

Preparing for sleep

The time leading up to sleep is very important. Build in a **wind-down** time in the evening when you are less active. Physical over-activity such as exercising, or eating too much just before bed, can keep you awake. Even rushing to get chores done for the next day can over-stimulate you and affect sleep. Sometimes people read or watch television while lying in bed. This may help them wind down, but for many people it can make them become more alert and add to sleep problems.

Am I engaging in activities which wake me up when I should be winding down?

Yes ☐ No ☐

If you answered 'yes', keep your bed as a place for sleep or sex. Don't lie on your bed reading, watching TV, working or worrying. This will only wake you up and prevent you from sleeping. You need to decide whether listening to a radio or music helps you sleep or not. Don't exercise in the half-hour before going to sleep as it may wake you up.

What about caffeine?

You have already read about the impact of caffeine earlier in this workbook. Caffeine is a chemical found in coffee, tea, cola drinks, hot chocolate and some herbal drinks. You have already found out that it causes increased alertness, however caffeine also reduces sleep quality. There is a real risk that a vicious circle can occur. Here the tiredness causes the person to drink more coffee to keep alert. Then the coffee itself affects the person's sleep and worsens the original tiredness.

Am I drinking too much caffeine?

Yes ☐ No ☐

If you answered 'yes', caffeine-containing drinks should be reduced if you are drinking them to excess. If you regularly drink more than five cups of strong coffee a day, try to reduce your total caffeine intake. Do this in a step-by-step way, or switch slowly to decaffeinated coffees, cola or teas. Definitely avoid having a cup of coffee or a last cigarette before sleep. Both caffeine and nicotine will keep you awake. Some people find that a warm, milky drink can help them get off to sleep.

What about alcohol?

Sometimes people drink alcohol to reduce feelings of tension and help get off to sleep. One unit of alcohol is about half a pint of beer, one measure of spirits or one glass of wine. Note that the strength of wine, spirits, etc. varies so this is an approximate summary only. It is suggested that women don't have more than 2–3 units a day, and men 3–4 units a day. If you drink more than the recommended levels of alcohol (22 units a week for women and 28 units for men), this can cause problems such as anxiety, depression and sleeplessness. Longer-term high levels of drinking also can cause physical problems such as ulcers and liver damage, and affect your relationships and work. Finally, drinking too much will cause you to go to the toilet more than usual at night. This will keep you awake.

Am I drinking too much alcohol?

Yes ☐ No ☐

If you answered 'yes', getting up in the night to use the toilet can be avoided by reducing the amount you drink before going to bed. If you take a diuretic (a water tablet), you should aim to take these earlier in the day. Discuss this with your doctor. If you drink above the **healthy drink range**, try to cut down the amount in a slow step-by-step manner. Discuss how best to do this with your healthcare practitioner.

An additional book providing you with practical ideas to reduce drinking (*Fix your drinking problem in 2 days*) is available from www.fiveareas.com.

What about your sleep pattern?

If you are not sleeping well it can be tempting to go to bed either *very much earlier* or *very much later* than normal. **Napping** is another habit that can end up backfiring by upsetting the natural sleep–wake cycle.

Do I have a disrupted sleep pattern (time to bed/getting up)?

Yes ☐ No ☐

If you answered 'yes', set yourself regular sleep times. Get up at a set time even if you have slept poorly. Try to teach your body what time to fall asleep and what time to get up. Go to sleep some time between 10 pm and midnight. Try to get up at a *sensible* time between 7 am and 9 am. Adjust these times to fit your own circumstances. When you cannot get off to sleep, do an activity until you feel 'sleepy tired', and then return to bed.

Tossing and turning in bed and clock-watching

Do you find yourself lying awake in bed tossing and turning, waking your partner up to talk ('... are you awake?') or just watching the clock?

Yes ☐ No ☐

If you answered 'yes', get up out of bed if you are not sleeping after 30 minutes. Go downstairs and do something else until you are 'sleepy tired' again. Then return to bed.

Area 5: Feelings

A range of different emotions can be linked to sleeplessness.

Do I feel anxious when I try to sleep?

Yes ☐ No ☐

If you answered 'yes', anxiety is a common cause of sleeplessness. It is often associated with a triggering of the body's **fight or flight adrenaline response**. This can cause the person to feel fidgety or restless. You may notice physical symptoms such as an increased heart rate, breathing rate, a churning stomach or tension throughout the body. The anxiety therefore acts to keep you alert. This is the opposite of what you want when you are trying to fall off to sleep.

Am I feeling upset or low in mood and no longer enjoying things as before?

Yes ☐ No ☐

If you answered 'yes', low mood and depression is a common cause of sleeplessness. For example, a person who is feeling down may find that it takes them several hours to get off to sleep. They may wake up several hours earlier than normal feeling unrested or on edge. Treatment of low mood can often be helpful in improving sleep.

Other emotions such as shame and anger can also be linked with sleeplessness.

Task

Look at the Five Areas assessment diagram below. Write in all the factors you have identified that affect you. These are possible targets for change.

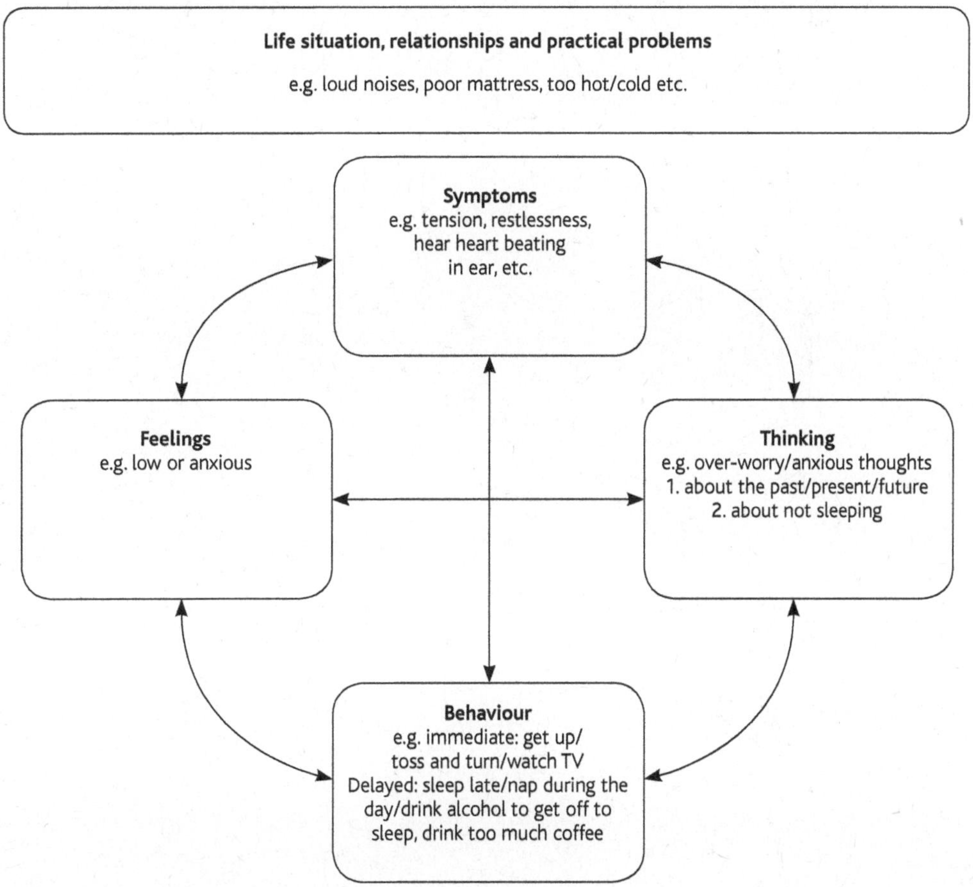

My Five Areas assessment of insomnia.

Overcoming sleeplessness

The treatment of insomnia involves two main steps:

1 Identify and challenge any anxious worrying.

2 Identify and reduce any unhelpful behaviours that are worsening your sleeplessness.

Your Five Areas assessment will have helped you to identify the problems you currently face and provided you with hints and tips in each of the main problem areas.

SECTION 5: Conclusion

Sleep problems are common. Treatment involves setting up helpful sleep patterns and challenging any anxious thoughts that act to worsen the problem.

Putting what you have learned into practice

- Try to get into a **routine**. Go to bed and get up at a regular time. Don't drink too much coffee, tea, hot chocolate and cola drinks, which contain caffeine. Around five cups or glasses a day of caffeine-containing drinks should be the maximum. Switch to decaffeinated drinks or water for drinks beyond this.
- **Nicotine** in cigarettes causes sleeplessness. Don't smoke just before bed.
- **Don't nap** during the day. It upsets your body clock.
- Watch your **alcohol** intake. Alcohol causes sleep to be shallow and unrefreshing. It also can make you wake up more to use the toilet.
- Consider the **surroundings** (noise, light levels, temperature and also the comfort of your bed).
- If you don't get off to sleep, **get up and leave your bedroom** until you feel 'sleepy-tired'. Then return to bed.

Don't expect to change everything immediately. However, with practice you can make helpful changes to your sleep pattern. If you have difficulties just do what you can.

My current goal

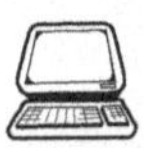

You can get additional help and support in problem solving at www.livinglifetothefull.com

Acknowledgements

The use of the Five Areas assessment model and associated language is used from the Overcoming Five Areas series by permission of Hodder Arnold Publishers and Dr C Williams. Illustrations are by Keith Chan and are reproduced with permission.

My notes

Toolbox E

Illness, symptoms and other people

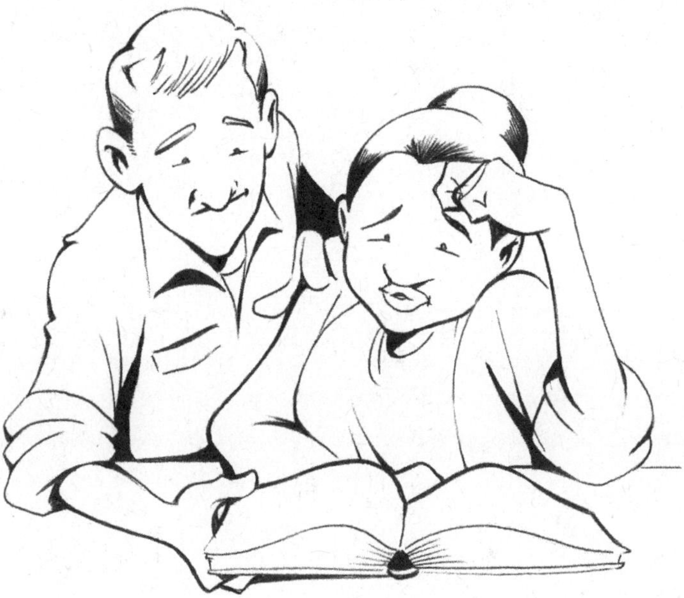

overcoming
functional neurological symptoms:
A Five Areas Approach

SECTION 1: Introduction

This workbook is aimed at not only at the person experiencing functional neurological symptoms but is particularly focused on those important family and friends around them. It summarises the key elements of the Five Areas Approach so that family and friends can understand and offer support in the best possible way.

In this workbook you will learn about:

- **What this course is about – and how the person is using it.**
- **How best to help and communicate effectively.**
- **Identifying helpful and unhelpful responses and learning ways of offering effective support.**
- **Looking after yourself and staying well.**
- **Putting what you've learned into practice in how you feel and what you do.**

Background for friends and family

The course workbooks use a proven approach based on cognitive behaviour therapy (a kind of talking therapy). Cognitive behavioural therapy is an effective form of treatment that can be helpful for people with functional neurological symptoms. Usually people would have a healthcare practitioner to help them work through this process, so you might have to take on the role of a supporter to the person you know with functional neurological symptoms. When symptoms have ground people down for a long time it can be hard to be objective both about the current situation and about how things were in the past. Your role as a supporter is to provide some of the information that is currently closed off to the person and to help them be objective and view the situation overall, and not just focus on the really difficult parts.

The approach helps us look in detail at five key areas of life. The **Five Areas assessment** provides a clear summary of the range of difficulties a person may face in each of the following areas:

1 Life situation, relationships, practical problems and difficulties (that is, the people and events around you)

2 Symptoms in the body.

3 Altered thinking (with extreme and unhelpful thinking).

4 Altered feelings (also called moods or emotions).

5 Altered behaviour or activity levels.

What a person thinks about a situation or problem may affect how they feel emotionally and physically. It also alters what they do.

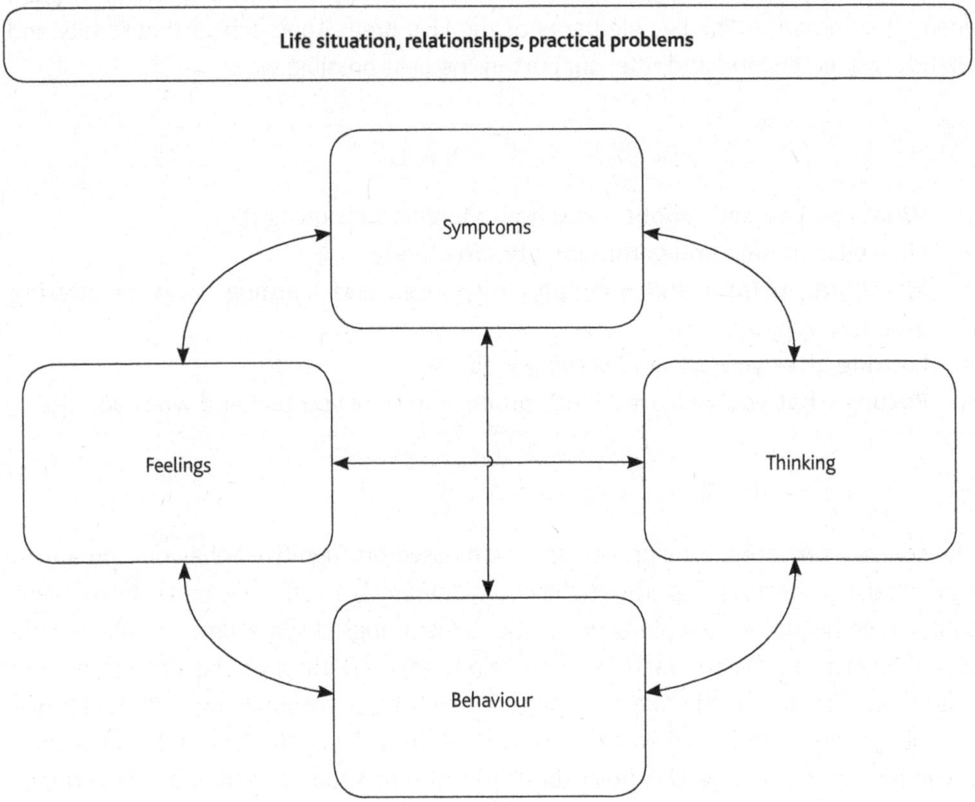

Because of the links between each of the areas, the actions that we take can worsen or keep our symptoms going. Importantly, it also means that helpful changes in any one of the areas can lead to benefits in the others as well.

About the workbook approach

The workbooks aim to help people bring about change in these five key areas. They are practical workbooks, which involve stopping, thinking and reflecting on the impact symptoms can have. They also teach key changes that can make a difference.

SECTION 2: How you can help

All of us are surrounded by people – and have all sorts of different friendships and relationships. The most important relationships are often with those people we either live with, or have a lot of contact with – such as friends, family members, partners, husbands and wives. When someone you know develops symptoms it can sometimes feel difficult knowing how best to help. Their symptoms can affect you too.

You may also be concerned about the reactions of other people to your friend's or relative's problem. For example, the attitude and comments of colleagues, bosses, healthcare practitioners, other friends or relatives, etc.

Ideally, we all want to be able to count on others to support us when ill. Sometimes however, we just don't know how best to help. Friends and relatives often (but not always) offer support when someone becomes ill. For example, in cases of flu, others may help by cooking food, helping with child care and doing the ironing. If an illness lasts for a number of weeks, months or years, you may find that this is difficult to keep up. Sometimes you may not know how to respond or offer support beyond short-term flowers and Get Well cards. Even when you try to help, you can be uncertain how best to do this. You may struggle to know what to say. If you feel like this you may be tempted to avoid talking about the symptoms and can even avoid visiting as a result.

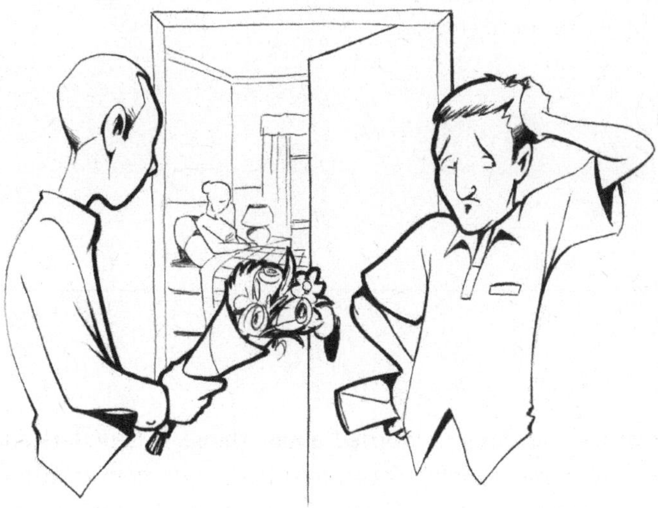

Where the illness isn't 'obvious' or always believed

When illness leads to a broken leg, there is a large plaster cast on the leg to see. Similarly with a chest infection the person will have lots of green phlegm to cough into little pots by their bedside. In cancer or heart disease there is a clearly diagnosed disease. Sometimes in functional neurological symptoms there is a clearly visible physical symptom – such as weakness, paralysis, etc. However some symptoms are not so visible, for example problems of tiredness, tingling, weakness, dizziness and pain. Sometimes the problem is simply that people (including some doctors) just do not know much about functional neurological symptoms. These problems are equally real. However, because they are less obvious sometimes the reaction of others may be less supportive. Part of this reflects difficulties others may have in understanding illness.

Checklist: Identifying some common problems that can arise for the person facing symptoms

They can't really talk and receive support from others.	Yes ☐	No ☐
There is no one around who they can really talk to.	Yes ☐	No ☐
Is anyone they know unsure about how best to offer support?	Yes ☐	No ☐
Has anyone begun to drop away from offering them support?	Yes ☐	No ☐
Are people around them avoiding talking about the symptoms and their impact?	Yes ☐	No ☐
Are the involved healthcare practitioners able to offer the kind of support needed?	Yes ☐	No ☐
Do they have symptoms that aren't 'visible' and obvious to others?	Yes ☐	No ☐
If they would answer 'yes', does this seem to affect how others react?	Yes ☐	No ☐
Write in what you have noticed here:		

The vicious circle of avoidance

When a person feels anxious or worried about things it is understandable that they tend to avoid situations, people, places, events or even conversations that they feel may be difficult or stressful. This avoidance adds to their problems because although they may feel less anxious or unwell in the short term, in the longer term such actions worsen the problem. A **vicious circle of avoidance** may result. The problem with avoidance is that it teaches people the unhelpful rule that the only way of dealing with a difficult situation is through avoiding it. The avoidance also reduces the opportunities to find out that the worst fears do not occur. It therefore worsens anxiety and further undermines people's confidence. The process is summarised in the diagram.

Example: David and Anne

David is in his 60s and has fatigue and problems walking. David's wife Anne has been very supportive and has taken on most work in the house and garden for over a year. She is now beginning to struggle and is feeling angry at David. He has changed so much from the man she once knew. He now sits in his chair watching television and hardly goes out at all. Anne is becoming embarrassed whenever friends ask her how he is. She is also ashamed about how angry she feels towards David at times. As a result, Anne is spending more and more time out of the house. She has become active in various local groups and when she is in tends to spend more time alone in the kitchen or the garden. David and Anne rarely talk and are drifting apart.

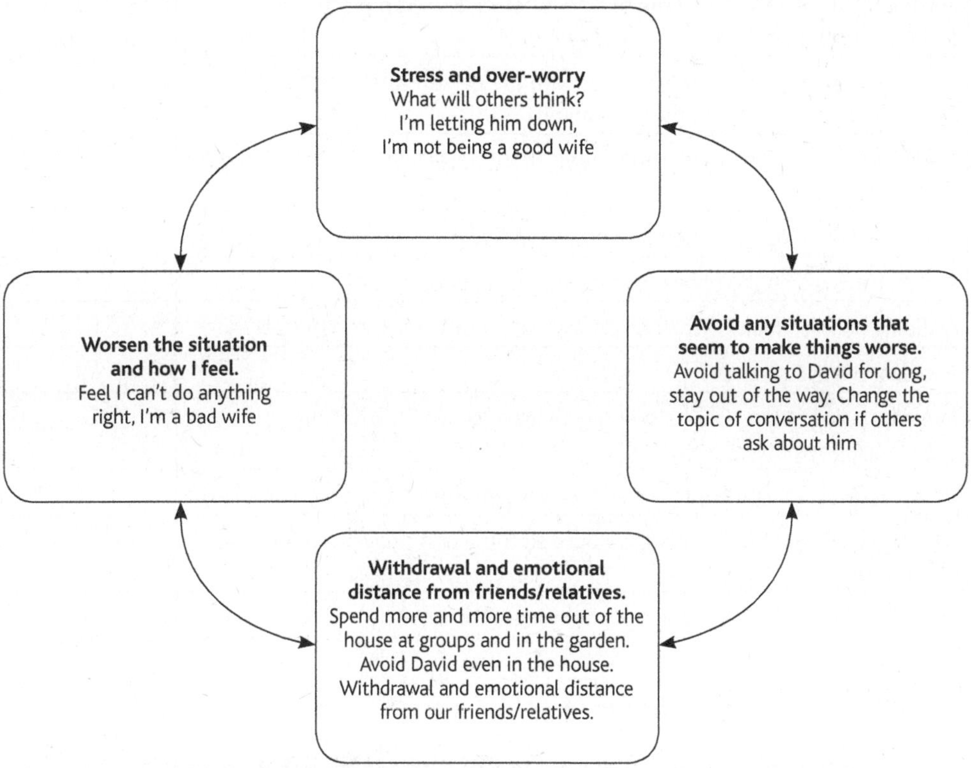

The vicious circle of avoidance: David's wife, Anne.

Sometimes, even just *talking about the symptoms* can become a topic that is avoided at home or with friends. This can backfire because others may be misinformed and misunderstand – in which case their imaginations may go into overdrive. Misinformation and rumour can actually create problems of gossip at work or among your neighbours.

Also even among closer relatives and friends, there may be an embarrassment over discussing things.

Task

The checklist below describes common areas of avoidance among families and friends. If avoidance is a problem, it is likely that there will be examples of avoidance in at least some of these areas.

Checklist: Identifying the vicious circle of avoidance

As a friend/family member, am I:	*Tick here if you have noticed this*
Avoiding talking to others about the symptoms?	☐
Putting off all decisions until the person is better. For example, putting holidays or other life plans completely on hold?	☐
Not really being honest with others or with the person with symptoms. For example, saying yes when I really mean no?	☐
Trying hard to avoid situations that bring about upsetting thoughts/ memories?	☐
Brooding over things and therefore no longer living my own life to the full?	☐
Avoiding answering the phone, or the door when people visit?	☐
Avoiding people/isolating the person with symptoms/us from others?	☐
Avoiding being assertive?	☐
Avoiding going out in public either by ourselves or with the person experiencing symptoms?	☐
Completely avoiding asking the person with symptoms about their problem?	☐
Avoiding being at home: keeping so busy so that I don't have to think about the problem?	☐
For partners/spouses: Avoiding sex or physical intimacy?	☐

Am I avoiding things in other ways?

Write in here how you are doing this if this is applicable to you.

To see if this applies to you ask, 'What have I/you stopped doing because of the symptoms?' Think about whether the vicious circle of avoidance applies to your situation.

Remember that at times the avoidance can be quite *subtle*. For example, choosing to steer conversations away from difficult areas that would actually benefit from being discussed.

Overcoming avoidance with clear communication

The only way of overcoming this is openness and honesty – and without this many problems can arise. If you are a person who worries about hurting other people's feelings, or aren't quite sure how to discuss these things openly, you would find it helpful to read Toolbox C (How to be more assertive).

You may find it helpful to make changes slowly. You could:

- Choose to spend more time together.
- Start to invite others round.
- Go out together if you can.
- Talk to each other – and listen, even if this is difficult.
- Find common ground even if you feel you have drifted apart.
- Make a joint decision about the level of information to give others about the symptoms. For example, deciding together on a simple one line reply. 'Things are much the same/going well' might be enough for most situations.

Here are some practical phrases and strategies you can use to relate differently to each other.

- 'This is obviously not a good time to talk, let's talk about it later.'
- Sometimes people need to work through an issue by talking at length. Let them talk, often no comment is needed. Listen for the main message, and then pick up on this point so the person knows you are really listening. For example, 'It sounds like you feel frustrated today ...'
- Offer praise and encouragement to build confidence, e.g. 'I can see such a difference from a month or so ago ...'
- Actively look for things you can comment positively about.
- Try to find at least three positive things to say every day.

KEY POINT

Children may have all sorts of unrealistic fears about possible outcomes if they are kept in the dark, so aim to keep communication clear. Here a child may worry that they have caused the problem, or fear that their parent or sibling may die, or go away, as a result of the symptoms. Take time to talk at the right level to your child in ways they understand. Several good books are also available to help children understand about symptoms.

SECTION 3: Family and friends: Helpful and unhelpful responses

When someone you care about needs your help, you often try to improve things for him or her through a range of actions. These might include a range of *helpful* responses, but also some *unhelpful* responses.

This section of the workbook focuses on the helpful and unhelpful behaviours that you as friends/relatives/carers may do.

Helpful activities by families and friends

- Finding out about the problem – through reading workbooks in this course, and asking healthcare practitioners. This can help equip you with the knowledge and skills you need.
- 'Being there' for the person for the long term.
- Being willing to talk and offer support when needed.
- Encouraging the person to put what they are learning in this course into practice.
- Keeping a positive but realistic outlook that change is possible but will take time. Realising there are no quick fixes.
- Using your sense of humour to cope.
- Planning time for you as well as for others.
- Using effective coping responses such as relaxation techniques (see Toolbox D) to deal with feelings of tension.
- Seeing a healthcare practitioner for advice if you yourself feel down/depressed.

Am I doing any other helpful behaviours?

Write in what you are doing here if this applies to you.

By planning to boost these helpful activities, this can improve how you and those around you feel.

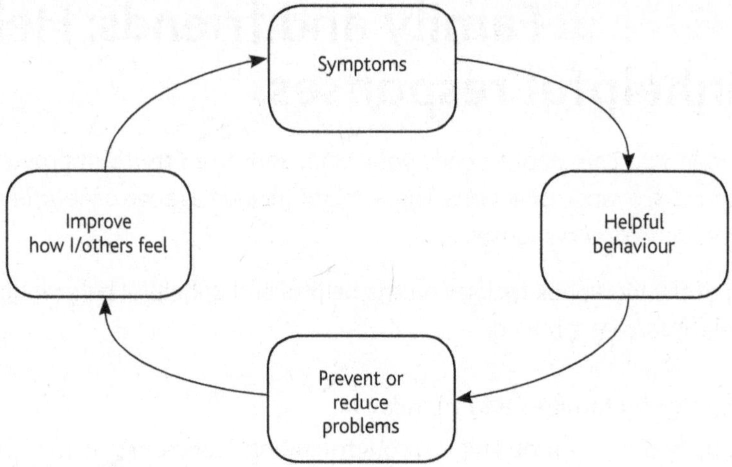

The circle of helpful behaviour.

Unhelpful behaviours by our family and friends

Sometimes, friends or family can act in ways that worsen the situation. These actions often make people feel better in the short term. However, they can also backfire and create further problems. For example, raising the voice in frustration can make a person feel a lot better to begin with. However, it can have a damaging effect on relationships and leave them feeling guilty. The results of unhelpful behaviours include immediate or longer-term problems. These actions therefore become part of the problem. A **vicious circle of unhelpful behaviour** may result. Other examples of unhelpful behaviour are:

- Offering 'helpful advice' all the time.
- A desire to do *everything* for the person.
- Constantly offering reassurance that everything will work out fine.
- Overly protecting and suffocating the person by taking away all their responsibility (and all their choices too).

There can be many reasons for family or friends to behave in this way. Often, it's due to concern, friendship and love. Sometimes it may be the result of anxiety, or occasionally guilt. Whatever the cause, when others offer too much help and want to do everything for someone else, their actions can backfire in several ways.

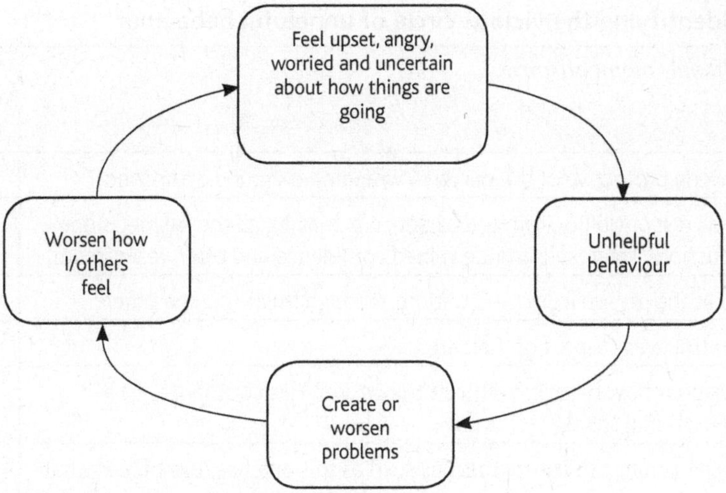

The vicious circle of unhelpful behaviour.

Frustration and anger at healthcare practitioners

When someone takes on a supportive or carer role, it's common to sometimes struggle. Different feelings such as demoralisation, worry, guilt, frustration or even anger can occur. These frustrations can spill over into how you talk about healthcare practitioners. It can be tempting to become critical and have very jaundiced views of doctors. Most healthcare practitioners are able to offer helpful support to people. However, from time to time even those working in the caring professions may not be as good at offering the kind of support that you feel your relative or friend requires. But the danger is that you undermine the advice that is being given in an unhelpful way.

Look at the following list and tick any activity you have found yourself doing over the last month. A wide range of different unhelpful behaviours have been listed here to help you to think about the changes that are happening in your own situation as a supporter or carer.

Checklist: Identifying the vicious circle of unhelpful behaviour

As a friend/family member, am I:	*Tick here if you have noticed this*
Becoming overly protective of the person – wrapping them in cotton wool?	☐
Taking over all responsibility from the person, e.g. making all the key decisions with no discussion? The result is undermined confidence and often resentment.	☐
Having a go at the person from time to time, through frustration or anger?	☐
Trying to control every aspect of their life?	☐
Talking only about how hard and difficult things are? This contributes to a downward emotional spiral.	☐
Advising the person not to try approaches such as this one because of fears that it may do harm?	☐
Criticising healthcare practitioners – because they haven't been able to find a cure?	☐
Undermining/criticising advice the person has received from a practitioner?	☐
Helping the person to avoid doing things because of fears about what harm might result? For example, taking over going to the shops, driving.	☐
Constantly reassuring the person?	☐
Constantly asking about the symptom, which just draws attention to it?	☐
Introducing the person as X, who has this problem, rather than just by their name? You have started seeing the symptoms, not the person.	☐
Telling the person to avoid any physical activity or exercise as a result of concerns about their physical health?	☐
Speaking for/over the person in social settings, or in medical outpatients, etc? You tell their story rather than them letting them talk.	☐

Often these behaviours are carried out with good intentions, or as a means of feeling better yourself in the short-term. The problem is that in the medium- to long-term the responses backfire for you or the person themselves. For example, undermining their belief in their healthcare practitioner may prevent them from engaging in approaches that might help. Speaking for the person in social settings can undermine their confidence and make it less likely that they will feel able to tackle their problems.

Wrapping the person in cotton wool

Offering extra special attention and support can also become unhelpful – even if done with the very best intentions. The relationship may feel **suffocating and frustrating**. They can end up feeling treated like a child. Arguments and little irritations build up and are upsetting all round. Although you mean well, your actions can actually *undermine* *your relationship*. When trying to cope with symptoms it is important to encourage the person to keep as active as possible within the confines of how they feel. If you take responsibility for doing everything, the danger is that they are not as active as they could be and you create unnecessary dependency.

Example: Becoming overly protective

★ David has reduced activity and is worried by the long grass in his garden. His wife has banned him from doing any of the gardening – even though she is struggling to cope. They are paying a gardener and whenever David sees him he feels deep shame that he cannot do even this. His wife's well-meaning and overly protective actions have undermined how he feels.

★ Jane's colleagues at work have taken over buying stock on her behalf and as a result she can manage to avoid going to the supermarket. This seems helpful in the short term, however in the longer term it is preventing her from rebuilding her confidence and has had an unhelpful impact on her life.

Example: Fostering avoidance

★ Caroline copes really well with managing her symptoms. However Caroline's husband often *declines invitations for meals out and other social situations on her behalf* without checking first. He doesn't want her to feel under pressure to attend social events. By doing this he limits Caroline's ability to decide for herself. This is in part due to him being unable to understand why she pushes herself but his actions undermine her. She is now finding her social life is becoming restricted. Her husband does this with the best intentions, but just hasn't thought through the longer-term consequences.

Staying well

When you support others you also need to look after yourself and allow time and space for your own needs. **Depression and stress are very common among carers**. The danger is that you are so busy offering support that you have no time for yourself. Helpful responses here include:

- An open discussion of your own stress as an issue.
- Taking short breaks/holidays/weekends away with others.
- Planning 'me time' such as hobbies/interests/night classes into the day and week.

- Attending relaxation or stress management groups/classes or carer support groups.
- Seeing your own doctor to discuss the need for additional treatment and support.

Problem actions and activities you need to be aware of

Although you try to cope as best you can, sometimes some of the ways of reacting can backfire and worsen the situation. The following are among a range of common unhelpful behaviours that you can try to help you cope.

As a friend/family member, am I trying to cope by:	*Tick here if you have noticed this*
Throwing myself into doing things so there are no opportunities to stop, think and reflect	☐
Pushing others away and being verbally or physically threatening/rude to them	☐
Becoming very demanding of others	☐
Looking to others to make decisions or sort out problems for me	☐
Drinking more than I should to block how I feel	☐
Using medication differently to how it is prescribed to improve how I feel or help me sleep, etc. (For example, taking an extra dose)	☐
Eating too much ('comfort eating'), or over-eating so much that this becomes a 'binge'	☐
Trying to spend my way out of how I feel by going shopping ('retail therapy')	☐
Deliberately harming myself	☐
Taking part in risk-taking actions, for example crossing the road without looking, or gambling using money I don't really have	☐

The next section provides some hints and tips of ways you can begin to reduce any unhelpful behaviours.

SECTION 4: Breaking the vicious circles and building helpful behaviours

To successfully plan a reduction in unhelpful behaviours, or to increase helpful behaviours, you need to have a clear plan. This applies whether the intention is to tackle such problems in your own life, or in helping the person you care form such a plan themselves.

Do:

- Plan to alter *only one* key behaviour over the next week. Do this one step at a time until you reach your eventual goal.
- Produce a plan to slowly alter what you do in a step-by-step way.
- Ask yourself the **questions for effective change** that follow to check that the change is well planned.
- Write down your plan in detail below so that you will be able to put it into practice this week.

Don't:

- Choose something that is too ambitious a target to start with.
- Try to start to alter too many things all at once.
- Be very negative and think 'nothing can be done, what's the point, it's a waste of time'. Try to experiment to find out if this negative thinking is accurate or helpful.

Building helpful behaviours and reducing unhelpful behaviours

The seven-step plan can help you to plan to do things differently.

Think about how you can begin to tackle the problems you face in your own life. This may be either:

- To reduce any unhelpful behaviour.
- To build up a helpful behaviour.

SECTION 5: Summary

In this workbook you have discovered:

- **What this course is about – and how the person is using it.**
- **How best to help and communicate effectively.**
- **How to identify helpful and unhelpful responses and learn ways of offering effective support.**
- **How to look after yourself and stay well.**

Putting what you have learned into practice

Reflect on the seven-step plan and consider how you can:

- Reduce one unhelpful response over the next week
- Plan to build upon one helpful response this week.

My current goal

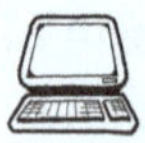

You can get additional help and support in problem solving at www.livinglifetothefull.com

Acknowledgements

The use of the Five Areas assessment model and associated language is used from the Overcoming Five Areas series by permission of Hodder Arnold Publishers and Dr C Williams. Illustrations are by Keith Chan and are reproduced with permission.

My notes

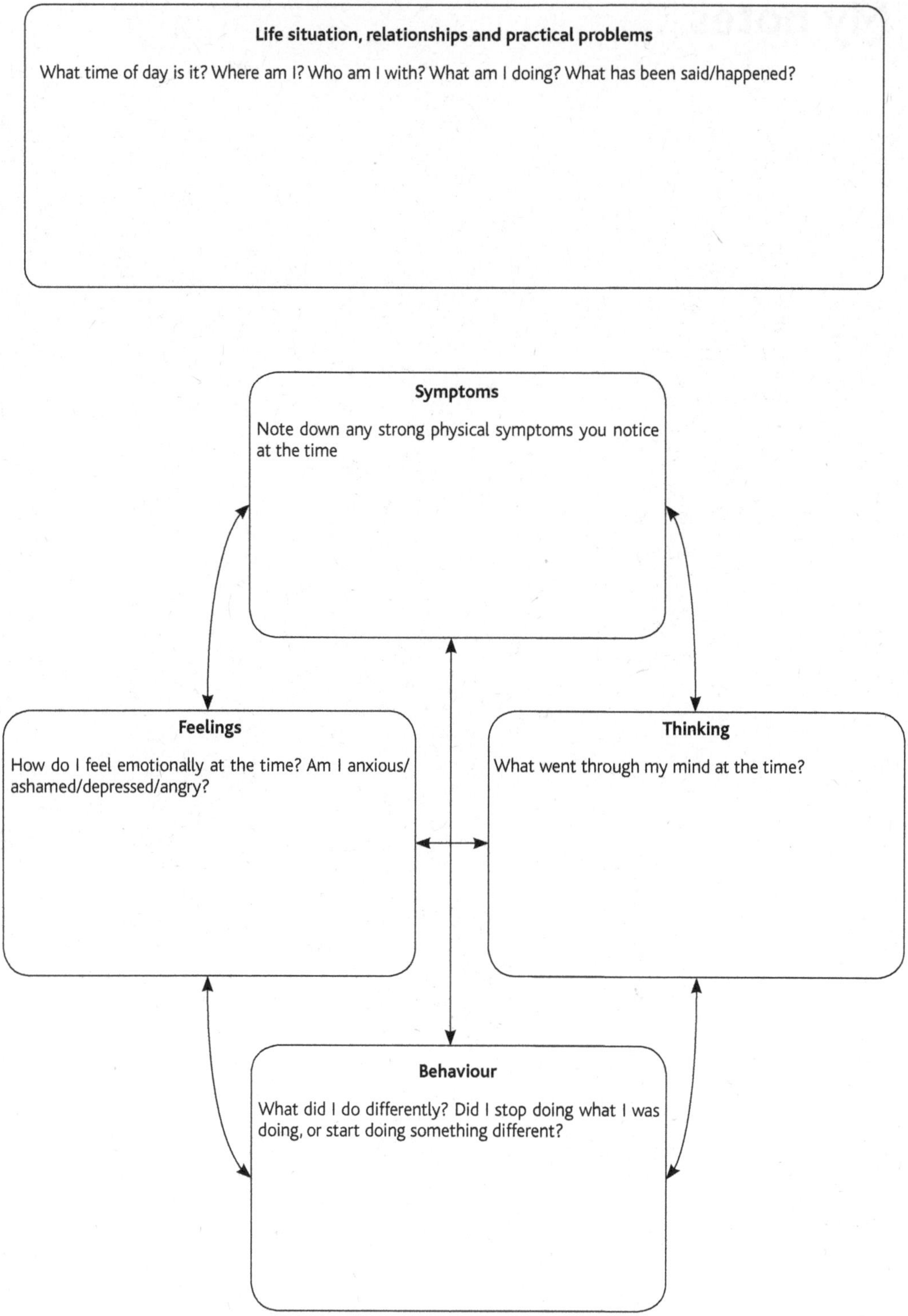

A Five Areas assessment of a specific time when I felt worse.

THOUGHT FLASHCARD: Noticing and changing unhelpful thoughts

Step 1: Think in detail about a specific time recently when you have felt worse

- Watch for a time when you feel worse, emotionally or physically.

Consider:

The time: What time of day is it? *The place:* Where am I?

The people: Who is present? *The events:* What has been said/what has happened?

Step 2: Identify your key thought: what went through your mind at the time?

You may notice several different thoughts.

- Choose the thought that is upsetting you the most: this is sometimes called the **key thought** as it is the key to understanding why you feel worse then.
- Overall, how much did you believe the key thought at the time? Mark with a cross or write a percentage:

Not at all (0%) ———————————— Completely believed (100%)

Step 3: Does the key thought show one of the unhelpful thinking styles?

- Am I being my own worst critic? (bias against yourself).
- Am I focusing on the bad in situations? (negative mental filter).
- Am I making negative predictions about the future? (gloomy view of the future).
- Am I jumping to the very worst conclusion?
- Am I second-guessing that others see me badly without actually checking if it's actually true? (mind-reading).
- Am I *taking unfair responsibility* for things that aren't really my fault/taking all the blame?
- Am I using unhelpful *must/should/ought/got to* statements? (making extreme statements or setting impossible standards)?

If you have answer yes to any of these questions, go to step 4. If not, stop here or choose another thought.

Step 4: How does this key thought affect you?

Does it worsen how I *feel* and unhelpfully alter what I *do*?

- Did it make me feel more upset?
- Did it stop/reduce me from doing something that would have possibly been fun/ given a sense of achievement? (reduced activity).
- Did it cause me to **avoid** particular situations, people or places leading me to restrict my life and undermine my confidence? (avoidance).
- Did it cause me to start doing something that ended up backfiring and worsening how I or others feel – in the short or longer term (consider the impacts on you physically, emotionally and on your relationships). (unhelpful behaviours).
- Finally, did believing the thought prevent you doing something helpful – like going out/staying active, etc.?
- Overall, did the key thought have an unhelpful effect on you?

Yes ☐ No ☐

Step 5: Stop, think and reflect on the key thought

Simply noticing the key thought and becoming aware of its effects may be enough.

- Label the key thought as *just another* of those extreme and unhelpful thoughts. These are just a part of what happens to most people in times of upset.
- **Allow the thought to be.** Try to take a step back from the thought as if observing it from a distance. Move your mind on to other more helpful things such as the future or recent achievements.
- Move on. Make an active choice to stay active/face any unhelpful fears/choose to react helpfully rather than unhelpfully

If this approach helps, then you can stop here. If you still find you are upset by the key thought go to step 6.

Step 6: Reflect on the key thought in more detail

It's easy to believe the worst when you are upset. Question the thought – don't just accept it. Is there anything to make you think the key thought is incorrect?

You might find it helpful to imagine you are in a courtroom demanding answers of the thought.

Use the seven key thought challenge questions – the questions the key thought doesn't want you to ask:

- What would I tell a friend who said the same thing?
- If I wasn't feeling like this what would I say?
- Am I basing this on how I feel rather than the facts?
- What would other people say? Have I heard different opinions from others about the same thought?
- Am I looking at the whole picture? Are there any other ways of explaining the situation that are more accurate?
- What would I say about this looking back six months from the future?
- Do I apply one set of standards to myself and another to others?

You may find it helpful to come up with a new *balanced and helpful conclusion* based upon your answers to these questions. Like a celebrity, key thoughts love attention. It's just not worth your attention. Allow it to **just be**.

Re-rate your belief in the key thought.

Not at all (0%) ―――――――――――――――― Completely believed (100%)

If this approach helps, then you can stop here. If you find you are still upset by the thought go to step 7.

Step 7: Experiment: act against the original key thought

It is important to decide not to be pushed around by the negative thought. A good way of doing this is:

- **Let it be** – choose not to turn it over again and again.
- Choose to **act against** the unhelpful thought. For example, if the thought says to you 'don't go to the meal, you won't enjoy it' – then go to the meal. If it says to you 'nobody wants to talk to me' – then choose to talk to someone and see how they react. If it says 'you can only cope if you drink/over-eat, etc.' – then choose not to drink or over-eat but instead respond more helpfully.

It may take time to build your confidence in this. The workbooks on overcoming avoidance, reduced activity and unhelpful behaviours may help you plan ways of slowly making these changes at a pace that you can cope with.

KEY POINT

Acting against your extreme and unhelpful thoughts will help undermine them.

Remember: This process takes time. With practice, you will build your confidence in using this approach.

You can also download additional worksheet resources free of charge from www.livinglifetothefull.com and www.fiveareas.com.